I KNOW I SHOULD EXERCISE, BUT...

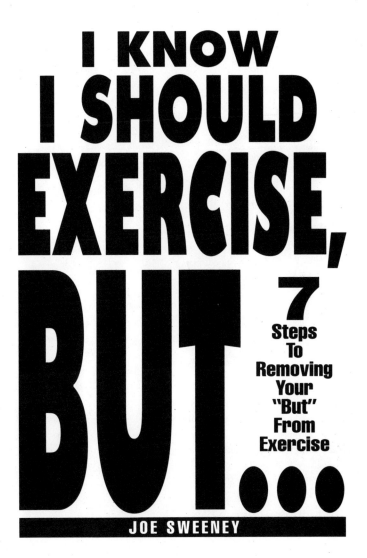

7 Steps To Removing Your "But" From Exercise

JOE SWEENEY

Foreword by Laura Walther Nathanson, M.D., F.A.A.P.

Pacific Valley Press
San Diego, California

Pacific Valley Press, Publisher
PO Box 927915
San Diego, California 92192-7915

Author: Joe Sweeney
Editor: Beth Hagman
Cover & Page Design: Beth Hagman
Author Photo by Pat Harrison
Foreword: Laura Walther Nathanson, M.D., FAAP

Library of Congress Catalog Card Number: 98-91780
ISBN: 0-9666163-2-4

Printed in the United States of America on recycled paper
First Edition

To my parents

Warning/Disclaimer

This book is designed to guide and motivate individuals toward a physically-active lifestyle. It is *not* intended to replace medical advice. **Check with your doctor before beginning any exercise program.**

Table of Contents

Acknowledgments

I appreciate everyone who helped me complete this book, including Mary-Ellen Drummond for her professional guidance and never-ending encouragement, Karen O'Connor and Mo Rafael for their valuable input, Pat Harrison for her photographic talents, and a huge thank you to Beth Hagman for her editing, page and cover design — and especially for her patience.

I also am grateful to mentor and friend Dana LaMon and friends Robin Bowman, Jim and Jill Turpin, Chuck Berke, Laura and Chuck Nathanson and Katrina Stacey-Hoeber for their frequent support and honest feedback during the various stages of the project.

Countless people have enriched my exercise experiences, including Deborah Emslie, Ernie Marinoni, Dolly Felix, Don Peckham, Herb Rose, Bob Wagner and Ron Sandvick. Also Susan Grant and Carson Kan — the charter members of our original hike-a-month club. I'd like to extend a special recognition to Alan Glover, the 'round-the-world bicyclist who inspired me to bike across the United States, and my late brother Tom, who persuaded me to pedal across the continent a second time.

My past years as a competitive gymnast continue to significantly influence how I view life today, so I thank my former gymnastics coaches Art Andrews, Clair Jennett, Nils Bengtsson, Dave Jacobs, Roy Davis, Bob Peavy and Rea Anders for helping me progress in that incredibly exciting and yet difficult sport.

Muchas gracias to Deborah Szekely, her son Alex and daughter Livia, General Manager Jose Manuel Jasso and the fabulous staff at Rancho La Puerta Fitness Resort for creating and operating the best destination spa I have ever seen. Thanks, also, to the thousands of spa guests who, over the past two decades, helped me form these seven steps to getting and staying physical.

Thanks to all of my past and present personal fitness training clients, in particular Linda Adams, Tom Gordon, Mahan

Missaghieh, Oscar Ruebhausen, Laura and Chuck Nathanson and Sandra Dijkstra, for their enthusiasm and willingness to work out consistently, and for their sense of humor— which helped them survive their time with me.

Congratulations to my sister Kath, who consistently follows her simple but balanced exercise routine and keeps her dog Popi in fine form at the same time. A reminder to my nephews Matt and Jeremy that I am confident I can still beat each of them one-on-one in basketball, as long as I cheat. To my brother Dennis, for coming up with the terrific suggestion to rendezvous in Yosemite and climb Half Dome. OK, Dennis, now that I've put that thought in print, let's get it done. Matt and Jeremy tell me they are ready. Perhaps Dianne, Teresa and Luis would like to join us, too.

About The Author

Joe Sweeney walks his talk. A lifelong exercise enthusiast, Joe began bouncing on a trampoline at his local Boy's Club at age eight. He later became a collegiate gymnastics champion (two-time Pacific Coast Athletic Association All Around Champion) and competed in five national gymnastics championships. During a fundraising event, he once performed 1,000 cartwheels in an hour.

When he retired from gymnastics competition, Joe filled the void with other physically-oriented sports, hobbies and adventures. In the 1970s, he piloted over 700 flights on a hang glider, including eighteen flights from Glacier Point in Yosemite National Park.

In the 1980s, he bicycled across America twice and once down the 1,000-mile length of Mexico's Baja Peninsula.

Joe has twice climbed Mt. Whitney, at 14, 494 feet the highest peak in the contiguous United States.

He has enjoyed numerous active vacations and expeditions, including trekking in the Lake District of England, kayaking in the San Juan Islands, bicycling in the Northeast Kingdom of Vermont, rafting the Colorado River through the Grand Canyon, tracking mountain lions in the wilderness of Idaho and hiking Mexico's Copper Canyon.

Joe earned a degree and teaching credential in Physical Education from San Jose State University. He has coached gymnastics at the club, high school and college levels and taught high school Physical Education.

Over the last thirty years, he has taught gymnastics, volleyball, hang gliding, board sailing, swimming, diving, soccer, tennis, walking, water exercise, weight training, stretching, yoga, frisbee, juggling and disco dancing. In that time, he guided more than 30,000 people, ages four to eighty-four, toward physical fitness and healthy living.

Although Joe has trained champion athletes, he is proudest of his work with novice exercisers, for they often exhibit the most enthusiasm and appreciation for physical movement, and they often make the most remarkable progress.

Since 1980, Joe has spent over 300 weeks as a speaker and instructor at Rancho La Puerta, North America's oldest fitness resort. At the world-famous spa, he has trained a wide range of people — including CEOs, entrepreneurs, housewives, athletes, couch potatoes, octogenarians, children and celebrities. While he has not been on the Oprah or Donahue talk shows, Oprah and Phil *have* been in Joe's exercise classes.

Today, Joe is an award-winning speaker who presents keynote addresses, seminars and workshops to corporations and associations on fitness, stress management and adventure. His clients include General Electric, NationsBank and the American Association of School Administrators. His most frequent presentation is: *How to Fit a Healthy Life into a Busy Life.*

Based in San Diego, California, Joe is also a personal fitness trainer.

Foreword

"This one's all used up. I need a new one."

That's what I said to Joe Sweeney a few years ago, in reference to my body. Well, not the *whole* thing — just the energy/strength/endurance part. Brave Joe, to become my personal trainer. My mother's idea of exercise was walking briskly to the nearest place where you could lie down with a good book. I inherited her genes.

If it hadn't been for the fact that my chosen field, pediatrics, is a contact sport, I might never have recognized the need to do something about this attitude. But I was faced with the daily demand for aerobics (chasing the little ones down the corridor), weight lifting (hoisting a reluctant thirty-pounder onto the exam table) and flexibility (crawling under said table to retrieve the thirty-pounder's twenty-pound sibling).

When I pointed out to Joe that I needed to become fast,

agile, and strong, but that I did not consider regular exercise an option, he merely smiled, like a person with superior knowledge.

This book contains Joe's program for getting you started exercising, enjoying what you do, and keeping you not *committed* so much as *entranced* with your new energy and delight in feeling good.

A big part of Joe's success is keeping the focus on fun. Like me, you may not be athletic, but you may be competitive. Perhaps you want to weigh in, preferably twice a day, preferably with a scale that reads into the fourth decimal place.

Listen to Joe.

"Don't focus on weight loss. That makes it feel like work. We're going to have fun. Sure, you'll get stronger, and you'll look better, and maybe you'll lose some weight. But what you really want to monitor is how good you feel, day by day."

Another part of Joe's approach is safety, which means *No Acute Pain.* (Yes, acronym lovers, this is the derivation of the word NAP.) It's easy for a non-athlete to get hurt in a brand-new exercise program. With Joe's guidance, you'll be fine. I know. I not only have stayed healthy since Joe entered my life, but cured a chronic shoulder and elbow problem. Indeed, I grew stronger without realizing it.

One day, there I was in little short-sleeved scrubs at a C-section, waiting for the baby to emerge. Suddenly the nurse next to me, who had attended deliveries with me for years, gave a little yelp. She was staring at my arm as if it had sprouted feathers.

"Good Lord, Dr. Nathanson!" she exclaimed. "You've got a Muscle!"

Ahh. That felt good.

You don't need Joe in your house as a personal trainer to take advantage of his ability to inspire and teach. Your key to becoming active and fit for a lifetime is shifting your point of view on exercise. Read this book and you will.

If you follow Joe's program, you may find yourself with a positively embarrassing amount of energy. For instance, all of a sudden I found myself writing a book about the importance of exercise for overweight children (*Kidshapes,* HarperCollins, 1994).

If Joe's philosophy can turn an inactive, fifty-something lady doctor/writer into a fairly good facsimile of a jock, and make the whole thing fun — think what his strategies can do for you.

Laura Walther Nathanson, M.D.

While maintaining a full-time pediatric practice, Dr. Nathanson has written two other books, *The Portable Pediatrician for Parents (Birth to Age Five)* and *The Portable Pediatrician's Guide to Kids from 5 to 12,* both published by HarperCollins. She writes a monthly column, "Ask Dr. Nathanson," for *PARENTS Magazine,* and is a contributing editor to the American Academy of Pediatrics publication, *Healthy Kids.*

As you read this book,

embrace a few strategies

that work

for you.

Enjoy your success,

then build on that success

by flipping through

the pages again

and implementing

more ideas.

Your Warm-Up

Do any of these excuses sound familiar? *"I don't exercise because..."*

- *I have no time*
- *I lack the motivation*
- *I'm not coordinated*
- *I always injure myself*
- *I'm too stressed to exercise*
- *I've never liked exercise*
- *I was always picked last in P.E.*
- *I'm too old to start*
- *I'm too tired*
- *I need to lose weight first*
- *I'm afraid I might become addicted to exercise*

I wrote this book to help you toss your excuses and get moving. Consider me your personal guidance counselor. I will show you how to begin an exercise program, how to progress safely, how to make it effective, how to stay motivated, and how to fit exercise into a busy schedule at home, at work, while on the road and during the holidays.

If you have never enjoyed exercise, I will help you learn to appreciate it enough to do it. You might even learn to like it. If you already work out regularly but often flirt with burnout, I will show you how to achieve greater balance and a fresh start with your exercise routine.

If you think you're too old to start, I'll tell you right now that you are wrong.

You need exercise more now than ever before. This high-tech world leaves you stressed. Your technology-enforced sedentary life stresses you further. Gone are the days when people hunted for their dinner. You don't even hunt for a phone booth anymore — you just reach for your car phone.

But there is good news in this modern world: No matter how long your list of excuses, you *can* become a regular exerciser. It doesn't matter if you never enjoyed exercise in the past, if you injured easily, if you have no coordination or if you were always picked last in P.E.

You *can* learn to get physical once and for all.

I know what it takes to be a regular exerciser. I've lived it. I've done it right and I've done it wrong. I have seen thousands of people get fit by following the right steps, and I've seen thousands of people fail by taking the wrong path.

The physical benefits of exercise are well known. Exercise can strengthen muscles and bones, decrease body fat, lower blood pressure and cholesterol and improve your defenses against heart disease, breast, uterine and colon cancer, diabetes, osteoporosis and arthritis.

Yet the promise of physical health or the threat of disease don't seem to be enough to get many people going. The American Heart Association now recognizes physical inactivity as a major risk factor for the development of coronary heart disease, yet only one out of five Americans engages in regular physical activity. Seek the *intangible* benefits of exercise and you are more likely to get moving — and keep moving.

• **Get active and your eating habits may improve.** As you begin to appreciate through exercise what your body is capable of doing, you may experience a blinding flash of the obvious: If you start fueling your body with higher quality foods, you might perform even better.

• **Exercise can help you quit smoking.** As you move your body, increase your heart rate and attempt to take some deep breaths for the first time in a long time, you become painfully aware of how smoking interferes with the efficient functioning of your heart-lung system. Annoyed by your wimpy level of stamina and endurance, you may become disgusted enough to quit your nicotine habit.

• **With regular exercise, you may not reverse the aging process, but you can slow it down.** Chronologically speaking, I am older than I was a year ago, but at the ripe old age of forty-nine, today I *feel* younger. I credit exercise for my youthful exuberance.

If you are ready to feel stronger and more vibrant, read on and get ready to enjoy your new-found energy and more youthful appearance.

Keep your photo I.D. handy — they may be asking you for it more often.

Three Common Fitness Afflictions

Before you learn and practice the Seven Steps to removing your "but" from exercise, you must learn to steer clear of three behaviors that can sabotage your efforts to get fit. I refer to these self-defeating fitness afflictions as *paralysis by analysis, perfectionitis* and *quickfixitis.*

• **Paralysis by analysis** is failing to take action on a subject due to over-examination. If you haven't started exercising yet because you are trying to determine the best exercise to do and the best time to do it, you suffer from *paralysis by analysis.*

• **Perfectionitis** is the belief that everything must be performed perfectly. If you think you must do sixty minutes of vigorous exercise every day, you suffer from *perfectionitis.* You can benefit from as little as ten minutes of exercise three days a week.

• **Quickfixitis** is the belief that an instant solution exists for every problem. If you hope to get fit in a week, you suffer from *quickfixitis.* You may need several weeks or even several months to get in shape. That's okay. As you will soon learn, your journey to fitness can be as enjoyable as your destination.

If you identify with any or all of these unproductive behaviors, you are about to do the right thing. The Seven Steps will help cure you of these fitness afflictions.

The Seven Steps

Soon you will learn the Seven Steps in detail and put them into practice. Here's an overview of each step.

• **Step 1** reminds you that exercise can and should be fun, no matter how negative an attitude about exercise you have had in the past.

• **Step 2** teaches you that when you slow your approach to exercise, you can actually progress faster. You will learn how to develop an effective pace.

• **Step 3** shows you the value of making plans to exercise and keeping those plans visible, how to schedule your exercise at home and while you are on the road, and how to take advantage of unplanned opportunities to move your body.

• **Step 4** teaches you how the support of friends and

events can help you develop more consistency with your workouts. You will discover ways to seek healthy support.

• **Step 5** teaches you how a balanced exercise routine strengthens your incentive to stay active. You will learn to identify and shore up the weak links in your workouts.

• **Step 6** explains how an active vacation can turn you into a regular exerciser for life. You'll learn about active vacation options, how to choose the right active holiday, how to prepare for it, how to get the most out of it and how to apply what you learn to your life at home.

• **Step 7** explains why, if you want to get active for a lifetime, *you absolutely must make exercise a priority*

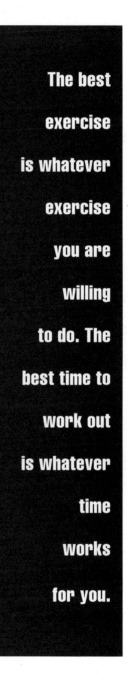

The best exercise is whatever exercise you are willing to do. The best time to work out is whatever time works for you.

in your life. If you think you're a long way from ranking exercise high on your life's list, don't worry. The first six Steps will gently steer you toward that big commitment, and Step Seven will take you over the top.

How To Use This Book

Read this book in an active manner. At the end of each page, sit up straight or stand up and stretch. At the end of each chapter, take a quick walk around the block.

When you come to the assignment at the end of each Step referred to as **Your Ten-Minute Solution**™, complete it on the spot and you will be ten minutes closer to leading an active life. The valuable ideas, concepts and examples in this book are worthless if you don't use them.

Since perfectionitis is not encouraged here, do not feel obligated to use every tip in this book. Some simply won't work for you. But be open to ideas that *might* work — even if they force you out of your comfort zone. As you move from step to step, try to embrace at least the *essence* of each step. Then modify the idea to fit your situation.

For instance, when I suggest that you devote ten minutes every Sunday evening to scheduling your exercise for the upcoming week, read "Sunday" as any convenient day. Whatever day you choose, however, stick with it — be consistent.

Expect **key ideas,** often supported by stories, examples, tips or quotes, to jump out at you in bold print.

Read every quote. They will inform, amuse, enlighten or inspire you. Quotes credited to JS are from yours truly (Joe Sweeney), but think of the initials JS as a reminder to *Just Start.* As you trek through this book, let *Just Start* be your mantra.

Follow the Seven Steps outlined in this book and you will succeed. You will get active, finally and forever. Follow the Seven Steps and you will never again utter that familiar phrase: *"I know I should exercise, but..."*

Note

✔ When I say "the spa" or "the resort," I am referring to Rancho La Puerta Fitness Resort, where I continue to visit several times a year as a guest instructor and speaker.

✔ *Beginner exerciser* refers to someone who has been working out for only one or two months.

✔ I will teach you two important number combinations in this book: 10-15-20 and 24-10-30. No, these are not locker combinations, but they *can* open doors for your fitness. Keep your eyes open for these powerful concepts.

If we were meant to move our bodies,

we would have been born with arms and legs.

—JS

Step 1:
Make Exercise Fun*

Mom was right.

Turn off the TV and go outside and play.

—JS

The question I am asked most often is, *"How do I find the time to exercise?"* I don't believe time is the real reason you don't exercise. Most excuses stem from unhealthy attitudes about physical activity. Maybe you look at exercise as a chore or a form of punishment.

If you think of exercise as an unpleasant task, no wonder you don't have the time for it! You probably don't have time to take out the garbage, either.

Choose activities you like. If you enjoy exercise, you will

*Check with your doctor before beginning any exercise program.

fit it in no matter how busy you are. Stop selecting an activity simply because it is trendy, all your friends do it or because it burns the greatest number of calories. None of those factors will inspire you to make a long-term commitment.

If exercise is such a pain that you need to offer yourself a reward to get yourself to move your body, then you have been approaching it all wrong. Exercise should be its own reward.

Say to yourself, "Exercise energizes me, relaxes me and clears the cobwebs from my mind. When I do an activity I like and at an intensity I enjoy, exercise is *fun.*"

Practice thinking, "I *want* to exercise." Put all your acting talents into it. You don't have to believe it at first — just say the words, out loud, as often as possible. If you catch yourself thinking "I *have* to exercise," stop right there and tell yourself, "No, that's wrong. I *want* to exercise." Visualize yourself exercising, laughing and enjoying yourself. This kind of mental reinforcement can make all the difference.

Once you've got your mind working for you, try some of the following suggestions.

Start With Walking

The body is built for action,

and the action for which it is specifically built

is walking.

—Aaron Sussman and Ruth Goode,
authors of *The Magic of Walking*, 1967

When it comes to exercising, you've got dozens of choices. If you're unsure where to start, begin your entry (or re-entry) into the world of fitness with walking.

Walking is natural, low impact, can be done just about anywhere, and the only equipment you need is a good pair of shoes. (Clothes are also recommended if you plan to walk in public.)

With walking, you can tone your muscles, relax your mind, heal or strengthen your back, improve your posture and have a good time. You can elevate your heart rate for an aerobic workout and, with proper technique (pumping your arms, pulling your heels underneath you and pushing off your feet), you can experience "a runner's high" while you walk — even on level terrain.

Talking while walking is easy, so you can socialize or brainstorm while you stride along. If you need to meet with someone anyway, take a walk and take care of business and exercise — all at the same time.

My grandmother started walking five miles a day

when she was 60. She's 95 now, and we don't

know where she is.

—Ellen DeGeneres

How to Walk

You may think you know how to walk — you've been doing it for most of your life. But there are a few things to think about if you're going to walk for fitness.

• **Walk tall.** Good posture helps you protect your back, breathe properly, look confident and feel good. Draw your abdominal muscles in slightly, lift your chest slightly, draw your shoulders back slightly and down. Imagine a string attached to the center of the top of your head, pulling you upward.

• **Keep your chin level with the ground.** Keep your

head up while your eyes gaze downward, looking for hazards — curbs, cracks in the pavement, dog poop and Elvis impersonators. No matter how short you are, you will appear tall if you walk tall.

• **Walk tall on treadmills.** Read the directions and get familiar with the display information before you start. During your workout, occasionally glance down at the data, but spend most of your treadmill time walking upright and forward on the belt.

• **Walk upright up hills.** Lean into the hill from the ankles. When you bend from the neck, back or hip, you inhibit your breathing, strain your back and miss the view.

Sometimes after the first day's hike at the resort, a guest or two complains

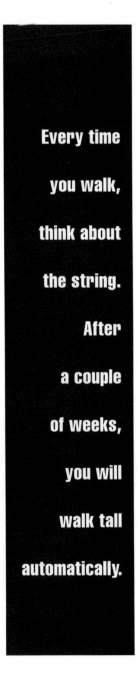

Every time you walk, think about the string. After a couple of weeks, you will walk tall automatically.

that their back has begun to hurt. I always ask, "Were you hunched over as you climbed the hill?" Usually, they admit they were. I tell them to think about the string, and that usually takes care of the problem.

- **When stepping up, keep heels down.** Plant your heel on the ground with each uphill step. Walking on your toes invites soreness and tightness in the calf muscles (those in the back of the lower leg).

- **Walk heel-and-toe on the downhills, too.** Walking heel and toe downhill causes less impact on your body than descending flat-footed. The rolling action of the feet distributes the stress on the body a little at a time.

I used to walk slowly down the hills when hiking at the fitness resort. Thinking I was protecting my right knee — which was sensitive to those dreaded downhills — I would shorten my stride and land flat-footed or on the ball of the foot with each step.

Despite my efforts (actually, *because* of my efforts), my knee got worse, not better.

Finally, I recalled the advice I had received years earlier

from a friend: *If downhill walking (or running) hurts your knees, try moving faster*. When I implemented that advice, my knee problem gradually disappeared.

Always maintain control on the downhills, however. If the descent becomes too steep or rocky to justify a fast descent, shorten your stride and slow down.

• **Walk without tension.** Walk heel-and-toe with a natural stride length and a natural arm swing (a pendulum motion). Relax your face.

• **Walk heartily.** When you're fit and ready to go faster, pump your arms. Bend your elbows at a ninety degree angle and drive each arm forward and back. Maintain a relaxed fist position, with the thumb and middle

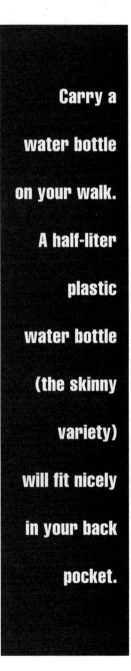

Carry a water bottle on your walk. A half-liter plastic water bottle (the skinny variety) will fit nicely in your back pocket.

> **Always keeping your arms bent can become a chore and take the fun out of walking. When you're not interested in walking fast, simply let your arms swing naturally at your sides.**

finger of each hand touching lightly. Keep your shoulders relaxed and down.

Then, *while pumping the arms,* pull the front leg underneath you and push off the toes of the back foot. The combination of working the arms with the legs will propel you forward faster and get more muscles involved—especially the heart muscle.

• **Breathe rhythmically.** On level terrain, inhale on three steps and exhale on three steps. If you're climbing a slope, your demand for oxygen will increase, so inhale on two steps and exhale on two steps. Walking up a very steep grade, you may need to inhale on one step and exhale on one step.

Breathe through your mouth to get ample amounts of oxygen to the muscles. Breathe fully, expanding your belly, ribcage and chest with each inhalation. Begin each exhalation by pulling your abdominal muscles in.

• **Walk against traffic.** When you must walk on the road, always face the car traffic so you can keep both eyes on approaching motor vehicles — and keep your workout from becoming a high-impact event.

• **Wear bright clothing.** Strive to be *seen*—not part of an accident *scene.*

• **Pass the talk test.** If you can't talk while walking, you're exercising too hard. Slow down.

• **Walk without hand or ankle weights.** When you walk with weights, you tend to slow down, and you don't get the high-intensity workout you hoped for. You also risk injury to your joints, your posture suffers and you definitely remove the fun.

Leave the weights at home and work your arms and legs instead. Savor the freedom of your unencumbered walk.

• **Walk before you run.** Starting your exercise program with running might be painful, and pain is no fun.

Become a walker first. Condition your body with a low-impact activity and later on you will be better prepared for a high-impact exercise such as running. You might even decide you can get an adequate workout with walking.

Give Footwear Some Forethought

Since feet do not come with a warranty, don't cheat on them. Invest in a quality pair of shoes — and socks.

Look for high-quality, cushioned socks that protect your feet from blisters, sweat and discomfort. There are styles specifically designed for walking, hiking, aerobics and other sports.

Your feet swell during the day so, for the best fit, shop for shoes in the afternoon. Wear the socks you intend to wear with your walking shoes and go to a store that specializes in athletic footwear. Speak to a salesperson who is also physically active. Tell them your intended weekly mileage and the type of walking you intend to do. Try the shoes on and walk around in them in the store.

Different shoes serve different purposes. For mall walking or walking on city streets, a walking shoe works great. For off road walking or hiking, especially on hilly terrain, a lightweight hiking boot or a running shoe with a waffle-type sole will work well. The more rugged the terrain you plan to cover, the more you'll benefit from the ankle support provided by a good hiking shoe.

Take A Hike

Why so many want to read about

the world of out-of-doors

when it's more interesting

simply to go for a walk

into the heart of it,

I don't fully understand.

—Edward Abbey

Marvel at the magic of hiking. You

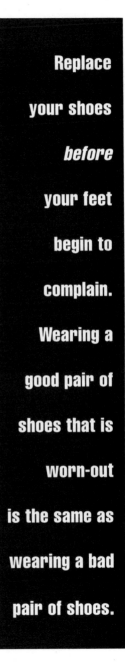

Replace your shoes *before* your feet begin to complain. Wearing a good pair of shoes that is worn-out is the same as wearing a bad pair of shoes.

Load your daypack with a book on birds, plants or animal tracks, binoculars (7x35s are great for birding), some snacks and plenty of water, and just let nature consume you.

become more trusting on a trail. When you cross paths with a walker on a sidewalk, you might not even make eye contact with the person. Yet, if you pass someone on a hiking trail, more often than not you will exchange a friendly greeting. That's reason enough to spend more time hiking.

You are guaranteed plenty of variety, every time you go hiking. For instance, the ever-changing surface of a hiking trail makes every foot strike feel unique. Walk on a natural surface and it feels like you are receiving a foot massage from Planet Earth.

I have hiked the trails at the spa over 1,000 times, yet I never get bored because no two hikes feel the same. The temperature, the wind, the moisture, the sounds, the smells, the texture of the clouds, the fog blanketing the valley below, the wildflowers, the birds soaring overhead, the rabbits scurrying for cover, the beetle executing a headstand in the middle of the trail or the spider web arching across the path... There's always something new, something I never noticed before.

If you easily get bored with exercise, go take a hike.

• **Dress in layers.** On a chilly day, dress so you're slightly cold to start. You'll warm up fast and start to peel off layers. Since you lose a lot of heat through your extremities, remove your hat and/or gloves — a quick way to cool off. If you begin to get cold, put the cap and gloves back on.

Add Pedal to Your Mettle

Riding a bicycle is another good, low-impact place to start your new exercise routine. Keep it fun and safe by doing the following:

• **Maximize your pedaling.** Whether you use a stationary or outdoor bike, put toe clips or foot straps on the pedals. Without some device to connect your shoes to the pedals, you can only push down. With straps and clips (or special pedals that enable your shoes to lock onto the pedals), you can push down *and* pull up with every stroke. You increase your pedaling efficiency, engage more muscles and reduce the pressure on your knees.

Before my first bicycle trip across America, I outfitted my touring bike with toe clips and straps to help protect my "bad" knee. Gradually, my knee got stronger. Two months and 4,000 miles later, I forgot I ever had a knee problem.

• **Keep the foot straps loose.** Unless you're competing in the Tour de France, *never* tighten the pedal straps on your outdoor bike. In case of a sudden stop, you need to be able to pull your foot out of the strap quickly. Even with loose-fitting straps, it's wise to practice pulling a foot out quickly and smoothly so, on that day when you suddenly stop, your foot is trained to exit the pedal strap and reach for the ground — so you won't fall over like a tree.

• **Bike early on Sunday mornings.** While the rest of the world sleeps, mount your bicycle on a Sunday morning as early as first light and enjoy a serene ride virtually absent of motor vehicles. It may take a bit of effort to get yourself out of bed but, as soon as you start your ride, you'll be glad you did.

- **Buy the right bicycle.** Know your purpose for purchasing a bike (exercise, rehabilitation of a knee, commuting, running errands, social riding, hill climbing, off road riding, competition, etc.) before visiting a bike shop. Tell the salesperson your purpose and your price range. Test ride a few models outside the store. Find a bicycle that fits your body and your intentions — those are the most important things.

"There are two kinds of cyclists: those who have crashed and those who are going to crash."

—Bob Wagner,
longtime leader of the Baja Bicycle Ride

- **Wear a helmet.** Recognize the risk of bicycle riding and be grateful that today's helmets are aerodynamic, lightweight and cool-looking. If you're being stubborn (and stupid), claiming your right to skip the helmet and increase your risk of cracking your head open like a melon, then consider wearing a helmet for the sake of your spouse or kids. Save your brain and set a fine example at the same time.

On Friday the thirteenth of May, 1983, I awoke in a hospital with no idea why I was there. I learned that one day earlier, while riding my bicycle, a car had hit me. I flew over the car's hood and landed head-first. Fortunately, the ground was there to break my fall. Although I suffered a concussion and amnesia from the accident, I eventually recovered (I think). My helmet did not survive; it had to be replaced. It did, however, serve its purpose well. Without a helmet, I'd be six feet under, or I'd be limited to one-syllable words while writing this book.

• **Use a mirror.** Can you imagine driving a car without a mirror? Most new automobiles are equipped with *three* mirrors! Unless you do all your riding off road, invest in a mirror so you'll always know what's approaching from behind (it's usually way bigger than you are).

You can attach a mirror to the handlebar, to your eyeglasses or to the helmet. I prefer the helmet or eyeglass mirror, since a handlebar mirror becomes useless if you're pedaling out of the saddle.

A bicycle mirror takes a little getting used to, but once you get accustomed to it, you'll never want to ride without it. In fact, you'll catch yourself glancing at the upper left hand corner of your forward vision whenever you hear a noise behind you... even when you're not on your bike.

• **Be bright.** Wear the brightest clothing possible and you increase your chances of being seen. Most motorists are not out to get cyclists, but they aren't looking out for cyclists, either.

• **Avoid night riding.** Period.

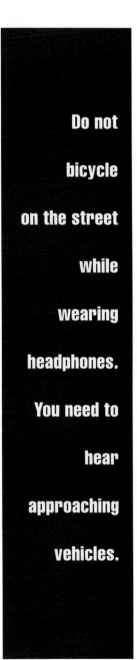

Do not bicycle on the street while wearing headphones. You need to hear approaching vehicles.

• **Bark at the dogs.** Yell at bicycle-chasing dogs louder than they bark at you. When Bowser approaches your bike, first glance ahead to be sure there are no hazards in your path. Then (while keeping both hands on the handlebars), quickly look at the dog and yell: *"Get outta here!"* or any phrase of your choice. What you say isn't as critical as how you say it. Sound as mean and nasty as possible, and never let 'em know you're scared.

Most bicycle-chasing dogs are not interested in chewing on your leg. They're either protecting their territory or they're out for a bit of exercise — with you as their personal trainer. The instant you yell, the startled dog will abort the chase. If it doesn't, you might have to repeat yourself.

Tempted to use your pump, water bottle or anti-dog spray? While spraying, you might collide with a car; your pump might end up in your spokes; and a mile after you deter the dog with water, you could die of heat stroke.

• **Tie a double knot.** Tie a double or triple knot in the shoelaces of your right shoe so they won't get snagged in your bike's chain.

Mix It Up

When you change your activity, you make exercise more fun for both your body and mind. For instance, walk one day and bicycle the next day. When you walk, you use primarily the muscles in the lower legs. On the days you bike, you work mostly the muscles in the upper legs, while your lower leg muscles take it easy.

Inserting different activities into your exercise program is known as cross-training. When you cross-train, you lower the risk of overuse injury, since different activities challenge different areas of the body. Meanwhile, you keep your mind exercised with a change of scenery. Cross-training makes perfect sense, because boredom and injury are two of the most common reasons people quit exercising.

• **Create your own endless combinations.** Alternate aerobics and weight training, or swimming and yoga. Or aerobics and weights and swimming *and* yoga.

Change the Character of Your Activity

Even without changing the form of exercise you do, you

Use objects or people to help you gauge your intervals. For instance, stride quickly until you reach the end of the block, catch that walker up ahead or pass that red pick-up truck in the distance. (I'm referring to the *parked* pick-up truck.)

can add interest to every workout by making small variations to your normal activity. Most of the following strategies will apply to walking as well as other types of workouts (running, bicycling, aerobics, swimming, in-line skating, etc.).

• **Vary your speed.** *(Disregard this suggestion if you are a beginner.)* Altering your speed will break the monotony of an even-paced workout.

For instance, after you are thoroughly warmed up, set the timer on your watch to sound every minute. When the alarm goes off, walk faster for one minute, then decrease your speed for one minute, then go faster again for the next minute, and so on.

• **Change the duration.** Lengthen or shorten your usual workout by ten minutes. Either way, both your body and your mind will appreciate the change.

• **Vary the slope.** Seek out hills and become familiar with muscles in your thighs and buttocks that you never knew you had. Keeping a steady pace up inclines will also strengthen your heart muscle.

• **Vary the time of day.** Change *when* you work out, and you will always alter your experience, even if your route and form of exercise remains the same.

✔ Enjoy the cool air and silence
  of an early morning walk.

✔ Stride and sweat in the warmth of a midday sun
  (pack water, hat and sunscreen).

✔ Marvel at the magic of a sunset stroll (take
  flashlight, jacket and a walking buddy).

✔ Visit your gym at a different time and meet new
  people.

• **Mix your company.** If you usually work out with a group, occasionally try it solo (as long as you know that you're safe). Working out alone, you will notice things about your body, mind and surroundings that conversations often hide. If you normally work out by yourself, invite a friend or two to join you, and enjoy the social interaction.

- **Vary the ground you walk on.** Constantly striding on hard surfaces is tough on your joints. To lessen the impact on your hips, feet and legs, seek out natural surfaces such as dirt or grass. Watch out for grass dotted with gopher holes and sprinkler heads.

- **Follow an easy day/hard day approach.** Vary the difficulty of your workouts from day to day, and you will have time to recover from your tougher workouts. With this approach, you can work out on consecutive days without overdoing it. For instance, plan a forty-minute brisk walk on Monday, a twenty-minute moderately-paced walk on Tuesday, a four-mile hilly walk on Wednesday and a two-mile easy stroll on flat terrain on Thursday.

Be Creative

Use your imagination, and you can turn a rather ordinary form of exercise into a real adventure.

I met a woman who pedaled a stationary bicycle across America. She bought maps of several states and, as she accumulated mileage on her indoor bike, she marked off the distance on her maps. She continued this odyssey during her resort vacation. Throughout the week people asked her, "Where are you?" By the end of her week at the resort, she was 200 miles west of Memphis, Tennessee — having a great time.

You could walk across your state on a treadmill, climb to the top of Mt. Everest on a step machine or row across Lake Michigan on a rowing machine. Sometimes the best adventures are only in your mind.

Don't Worry About Your Weight

When weight loss is your primary goal, you remove the fun from exercise. You overdo, rush and select activities you don't even like. Eventually, you become bored, exhausted, cranky or injured — and then you quit. Stay off the scales, and you'll have a better chance of staying on course with your workouts.

Judy has been coming to the spa for many years, and her daily routine during each annual visit is always the same. She climbs the mountain at 6:30 a.m., takes aerobics at 9:00, tones her muscles with rubber bands at 10:00, works her abdominals at 11:00, pumps iron in the dumbbells class at 2:00 and works her midsection (again) in the abdominals class at 3:00. Every afternoon at 4:00, she walks on the treadmill for an hour.

Unfortunately, Judy's level of fitness is poor and she usually struggles with the challenging classes she chooses. She's driven by a strong desire to lose weight during her spa week, and weighs herself two or three times a day. I often hear her complain that she is losing little or no weight.

One day, I asked Judy what she does at home for exercise. She snapped, "Are you kidding me? I don't exercise at home. I can't *stand* exercise."

Although Judy is an extreme example, I have met many people both at the resort and elsewhere with weight-loss-at-any-cost attitudes. Fortunately, I have also met plenty of people like Betty.

Betty arrived at the resort — not obsessed with rapid weight loss, but with a desire to find an exercise she could take home. During her second visit, Betty told me that her first spa experience had turned her on to walking. In the intervening year, she walked on a regular basis — and lost twenty-five pounds. At the same time, a back problem, which had bothered her for years, disappeared. She had no idea how that happened, but I bet Betty's year of walking helped correct her back condition.

Become a regular exerciser as Betty did, and you will probably lose weight, too. I say *probably* because, since muscle weighs more than fat, you could follow an exercise program for a few months and actually gain a few pounds.

I weighed myself just before I began my first bicycle trip across the United States. Eighty days, fifteen states and 4,300 miles later, after pedaling ten hours a day from California to Massachusetts, I flew home and stepped on the same scale. I weighed exactly the same as before.

Although the scale registered nothing, I knew that my body had changed considerably. I could tell I had gained muscle in my upper legs when, soon after my bike journey, I stepped into an old pair of slacks. They fit skin tight around my thighs — and loose around my waist. With a quick glance in the mirror, I could see that I had also trimmed fat from my midsection.

Incidentally, I felt great after the trip. Yet, if I just used the bathroom scale to gauge progress with my fitness, I might have turned a blind eye to my gains and concluded that I had just wasted eighty days of my life.

When people say they have lost five pounds,
ask them: "Five pounds of what?"

—JS

The scale does not distinguish between muscle, fat, water and bone, so save yourself the stress and stop placing so much importance on weight loss.

Stop managing your weight and start managing your health. Move your body consistently, follow a varied diet low in saturated fats and high in fruits, vegetables and whole grains, and you will be very pleased with your results. Without the scale to distract you, you'll notice how exercise enhances your mood and your emotions.

Exercise for Reasons Other Than Weight Loss

Regular exercisers don't dwell on weight loss. When I ask physically active individuals why they exercise, they say they feel an increase in energy and endurance, they are more mentally alert and better able to cope with stress. Weight loss is not their driving force.

• **Exercise for your mind.** Exercise helps you develop mental energy, confidence, discipline and focus — attractive characteristics that can enhance all areas of your life.

Although I spent three hours a day

If you must see numbers to gauge your progress, get your body fat measured. Ask your doctor or fitness facility about the appropriate tests. Repeat the test in six months, using the same method and the same technician as before.

training in gymnastics during my college days, I still managed to graduate in four years. The discipline I developed from athletics spilled over to my studies. I also developed the confidence that if I could do gymnastics, I could do just about anything.

• **Exercise for practical reasons.** Stay active so you can:

✔ Climb the slope from your mailbox to your house without getting out of breath.

✔ Clean out the garage on Saturday and still get out of bed on Sunday.

✔ Keep up with your children or grandchildren.

✔ Fit into your clothes — and be able to find clothes that fit.

• **Exercise for the social interaction.** Physical activity can serve as a great icebreaker. Bring a bunch of strangers together, get them involved in a game or sport and they won't be strangers for long.

As I arrived to teach 10:00 a.m. volleyball at the resort one Sunday — Day 1 for the spa guests — a man sporting a full head of white hair stood alone off the court with his arms folded across his chest and his head tilted down. I approached him and said, "Come on, Phil, let's play volleyball." Without saying a word, he followed me onto the court.

As I put the men through bump, set and serve drills during the next twenty minutes, Phil maintained his silence. None of the other volleyball neophytes were talking, either. Everyone was concentrating on the basic skills.

Finally, I formed two teams, with Phil on the team opposite mine. Early in the first game, Phil came alive — realizing that he was as skilled a player as anyone on his side of the court. At that instant, he became his team's self-appointed coach, captain, cheerleader and spiritual director. He started shouting encouragement to his teammates, talking strategy and exchanging high-fives.

Phil Donahue was no longer the reluctant participant. He was Mr. Volleyball. As I marveled at his rapid transformation from shy kid on the playground to team leader, I concluded that, some day, he might make a great television talk show host.

Your Ten-Minute Solution™

Before you turn the page, complete the following:

✔ **Call your doctor now to schedule a physical check-up.** Make sure it's safe before you start any exercise program.

✔ **Go for an easy five-minute walk.** Tune into how you feel during and right after your walk. How does the walk affect your energy level and your mood? During your walk, do not step in any potholes. After your walk, do not step on any scales!

✔ **Remove the bathroom scale from your life.** Convert your scale into a base for a potted plant or donate it to a high school wrestling program so the team can use it for their weekly weigh-ins.

Step 2:
Give Pace A Chance

There are no shortcuts to anywhere worth going.

—Beverly Sills

This is a quick-fix society. You want your oatmeal cooked in an instant, your film developed in an hour and your fitness in a day — a week at the most. You may be satisfied with how your hot cereal tastes and how your photos look, but you will suffer if you try to get fit too fast. You can't succeed with fitness if quickfixitis* rules your life.

If you wish to remove your "but" from exercise, you must start at a sensible pace and learn to keep to a healthy speed limit.

I was cured of quickfixitis at age 19. Midway through my

See Your Warm-Up, page 5

ten-year career in the difficult and dangerous sport of gymnastics, I heard a coach say, "The slow way is the fast way." At first, I didn't understand that expression. I guess I needed to fall on my head a few more times.

Finally, I got it. I slowed my approach to gymnastics and focused on the fundamentals for awhile. Suddenly, I realized I wasn't injuring myself as often, and I was wasting less time developing bad habits. When I finally attempted the advanced skills, I learned many of the complex tricks very quickly. At last, I was able to make steady progress.

The slow way truly *is* the fast way.

When I retired from gymnastics, I got involved in another high-risk activity — hang gliding. I applied my new "slow way" philosophy and, after six years and over 700 flights, I was still alive and well.

Unfortunately, I encountered many hang glider pilots who showed no regard for the slow approach. Nine of my friends and acquaintances died while hang gliding. All nine accidents were preventable, but the pilots were too anxious to enjoy the thrill of flight. One pilot, waiting for his new glider to arrive, continued to fly a condemned glider until he dove into the ground. Another pilot forgot to connect himself to his glider before launching from a cliff. The day I had to tell a pilot's wife that her husband had died, I decided to take a break from hang gliding.

Not long afterward, I climbed on my ten-speed bike and went for a leisurely ride in the Santa Cruz mountains. As I descended a long grade, a motorist recklessly sped past me, lost control of his car and crashed. While I helped the dazed driver climb out of his overturned vehicle, I realized that there is no escape from people who travel too fast in life.

Slow and steady wins the race.

—Aesop's Fables, *The Tortoise and the Hare*

The first time I visited the resort, I realized how few people practiced the "slow way" philosophy. Due to the short visit (seven days) of the typical guest, the tendency is to shoot for the quick fix.

My greatest challenge as a fitness instructor at the spa

remains constant: Keep people from doing too much too soon.

One day, while I was leading about fifty guests through warm-up exercises before the mountain hike, I noticed Oprah Winfrey in the eager group. She was not a fit woman at the time. She had yet to lose the infamous sixty-seven pounds that she would later symbolically wheel across a stage in a little red wagon on national television.

That first morning of a new spa week, I was hoping that Oprah would test her fitness on the meadow walk instead of on our steep and challenging mountain. I figured that if she over-exerted herself and had a health emergency, it would be bad news for Oprah and lousy publicity for the resort.

But Oprah was on a mission. She was to be a presenter at the Academy Awards a week and a half later and wanted to fit into a particular dress for the occasion. She had come to the resort to drop a lot of weight, and drop it fast.

Oprah made it to the top of the mountain that day, although I don't think she enjoyed the climb. She did lose some weight at the spa, and she did wear that outfit at the

Academy Awards. However, during the next few years, she gained, lost and regained weight numerous times. Finally, she realized fitness must be a lifestyle change and not a quick fix. The results of that decision are visible today.

An older and wiser Oprah admitted on her talk show, referring to her earlier attempts at fitness: "You can do it, but there are no shortcuts."

Be patient with your fitness. Just as the construction of a high-rise building accelerates *after* the foundation is in place, accept slow progress in the beginning while you lay your groundwork.

Ease into exercise, and later on you will enjoy a surge to success.

Use the 10-15-20 Approach™

If you have always been in a hurry to get fit, it's time to take a deep breath, slow down and follow the smart path. This method will get you there.

If you have not exercised for a few months, years or decades, or if you want to add a new activity to your routine:

✔ Begin with **10** minutes of low intensity exercise —
every other day.

✔ After two weeks, increase your workouts to **15**
minutes each.

✔ Two weeks later, expand to **20** minutes — every
other day.

Continue to gradually lengthen your workouts until you
are doing at least thirty minutes of exercise on most days of
the week.

Using the **10-15-20 Approach**™, you ease yourself into
exercise without causing pain or injury. Your early invest-
ments in exercise are small, but consistent. After only a few
weeks, your workouts will feel like a habit and as natural as
brushing your teeth.

One of the best reasons to start small: No matter how
busy you are, you have time for a ten-minute workout.

You may scoff at the notion that ten minutes of exercise
will do you any good. Yet, if you do it and continue with the
10-15-20 Approach™, those ten minutes could change
your life — for good.

A neighbor of mine asked me for advice on starting an exercise program. She admitted that she was in very poor shape, but she assured me that her doctor had given her the green light to start exercising.

I suggested that she walk for ten minutes at an easy pace every other day for two weeks, then at week three increase her workouts to fifteen minutes and gradually build to at least thirty minutes, every other day.

She smiled and said, "That's good advice; I'll do that."

She confessed to me a couple of days later that, during her initial walk, she wandered around the neighborhood for ONE HOUR! She was tired and sore afterwards, and did not enjoy her lengthy walk.

If you are a novice exerciser, end your first workout at ten minutes — no matter what. Play it safe. Make your inaugural workout a positive experience and you will eagerly await your next workout.

Worst of all, she did not work out again.

Avoiding pain is smart. When you are not distracted by physical discomfort, you are more likely to notice improvement. The moment you sense you are getting stronger, your motivation to keep moving will strengthen, also.

> *It is not important that you do a lot of exercise*
> *in the beginning. It is important that*
> *your exercise HAS a beginning.*

> —JS

Increase Your Incidence of Incidental Exercise

Brief bouts of exercise can be beneficial to your health and fitness. Sure, a thirty-minute workout is better, but three ten-minute sessions are worth it. The more often you move, even in small increments, the quicker you get accustomed to exercise and begin to develop momentum.

There are many ways you can add a little exercise into your life:

• **Park in the far end of the lot.** Finding a space will be easy, you will reduce the risk of someone's car door dinging the side of your vehicle — and you'll get a few extra brisk steps in.

• **Walk to the post office or store.** You avoid the hassle of parking — and you'll get some exercise. A bag of groceries carried on the way back even gives you a bit of weight training.

• **Step off the bus one stop early.** As you walk the remaining few blocks to work, the brief stroll will energize you and help you start your day.

• **Ride your bicycle to visit friends on the weekend.** Your friends are worth the effort, and your healthy example may influence them to get moving.

• **When you need to rest your mind, take a brief walk.** The movement will clear your head. Just a few minutes into your walk, you may suddenly grasp that clever idea that eluded you when you were velcroed to your desk.

• **Walk to release tension.** Ten minutes of walking represents ten minutes you are not slouched in your chair tensing your shoulders, rounding your back or straining your eyes on a computer screen.

• **Use more stairs and fewer elevators.** Stairs are much cheaper and just as effective as expensive gym equipment. Use them wherever you find them. Taking even a single flight of stairs will energize your mind and body. Arrive at your destination fully alert and ready for action.

• **Wash your own car.** As you bend, stretch, wipe and reach, you will use plenty of muscles in many different ways. Knowing you deserve the credit, you will be prouder than ever of your shiny vehicle. If you continue to take your car to a commercial car wash, however, take a walk while you wait.

• **Do your own gardening and yard work.** Get down and dirty and you will view your garden with greater pride than ever before. Vary your position frequently to lessen the strain on your knees and your back.

• **Retire the power mower and the gas-powered leaf-blower.** Dust the cobwebs off your human-powered mower and your rake and broom, and give yourself a total body workout without having to commute to the gym. Your neighbors will thank you for cleaning up quietly and for not blowing your leaves into their yard. Your body will thank you with improved tone and flexibility.

• **Read your mail afoot.** If you examine your mail while walking around your office or residence, you will tend to throw away those unimportant items instead of stacking them on your desk where they would only serve as a distraction.

• **Brush your teeth afoot.** Since walking upright is more comfortable than bending over the sink, you might increase your brushing time when you roam the house.

By the way, I do not suggest that you pace your house while flossing, unless you live alone—or you *want* to live alone.

• **Talk on the phone afoot.** Buy

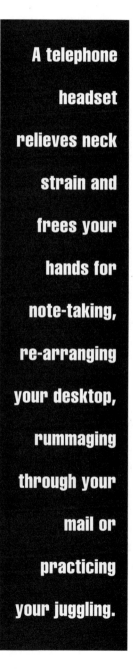

A telephone headset relieves neck strain and frees your hands for note-taking, re-arranging your desktop, rummaging through your mail or practicing your juggling.

a thirty-foot extension cord and walk while you talk. Your back and legs will enjoy the relief from sitting, and your voice will exude more energy.

• **Try Commercial Stretching**™. Since three things in life are certain — death, taxes and TV commercials — spend those commercial minutes stretching. **Commercial Stretching**™ is synergistic. If you repeat the same stretch during each break in a half-hour TV program, you will build on the flexibility you achieved during previous commercials.

At the first TV break, get moving by walking around the house for a minute. Then perform the following stretch for the duration of the commercial or until it's no longer comfortable (I'm referring to the stretch, not the commercial).

✔ Stand with your feet hip-width apart, your legs slightly bent and your hands on your thighs just above your knees. Inhale.

✔ On each exhalation, slowly draw your abdominal muscles in and up, while lowering your head and tailbone and rounding your back. Feel a stretch in the back.

✔ On every inhalation, slowly lower your belly and lift your head and tailbone, arching your back.

✔ Repeat several times.

As you repetitively move your back from a rounded to arched position, you release tightness in your muscles and spine. If you are a TVaholic, you will release some guilt, too.

• **Fidget your way to fitness.** Any amount of exercise is better than no exercise at all. Many people do not engage in any formal exercise, but they rarely sit still. Add activity to your day by seeking opportunities, no matter how brief, to walk, step, climb, carry, lift, dust, clean, wipe, scrape and scrub.

My parents, two active octogenarians, have kept in reasonable shape during their retirement years, not so much with formal exercise, but with fidgeting and frequent house cleaning. Dust is an endangered species in Michael and Dorothy Sweeney's house. Although they watch a fair amount of television, Mom and Dad are usually out of their chairs during the commercials — *doing something.*

Your Ten-Minute Solution™

Before you turn the page, complete the following:

✔ **List five low-intensity physical activities or physical chores,** each of which you could complete in ten minutes. Pick one of these activities and do it now.

✔ **List at least three pursuits in life** that demand a slow and gradual approach.

✔ **Add exercise** to the preceding list.

Step 3:
Plan to Move

"If you don't know where you're goin', you'll

probably end up somewhere else."

—Yogi Berra

If you intend to start exercising when you get around to it, you may never get around to it. Develop a specific plan to exercise and you will get your body moving. Plan to move and you will also succeed when most people exercise the least—on the road and during the holidays.

Schedule Your Workouts in Writing

On the same day each week (perhaps Sunday evening), list your exercise plans for the next seven days on your calendar or in your planner. Specify the day, time of day, type

> **List your workouts in red ink so they don't get lost in a sea of scribble. Each exercise session will jump out at you in bright, bold color, and you'll no longer say, "Gee, I meant to work out today, but I forgot."**

and length of each workout. Start modestly, with ten-minute workouts every other day. Treat each planned workout as an important item on your schedule and you will keep more of your fitness appointments.

Visible goals are easier to achieve. When I bicycled across America, I wrote my daily goals in map form. Each morning, I placed a map depicting a sixty-mile route atop my handlebar bag, and I glanced at it over a hundred times a day. Because my daily objective was in plain view and literally right under my nose, I always knew where I was going — and I usually got there.

It doesn't matter what your goal is. What's important is having a goal and scheduling it in. Write out what you want to do in each workout and post it where you will see it often, the night before and throughout the day.

Set a Challenging Goal

When you are exercising comfortably at the beginner level and are ready to take your fitness to new heights, select a goal for the month, the quarter or the whole year that is above your present level of fitness, but within reach if you train for it. Visualizing your long-term goal will be powerful. Those mental images will help you develop the greater resolve you need to stay consistent with your weekly workouts.

If you are a novice exerciser, planning to complete a 10K (6.2 miles) walk next month may seem frightening. Yet when you commit to that goal, you also commit to the training needed to accomplish it. A little fear can serve as a healthy source of motivation.

My friends and fellow speakers, Robin and Peter, decided to amass 1,000 miles of walking in 1996 — without selling their children or quitting their jobs. With a clear target in mind, they were able to cut a huge goal down to size. They knew how much they needed to walk each day, each week, each month. They always knew where they stood and were able to make adjustments as needed without losing sight of the big picture.

When I saw Robin and Peter in early February of that year, they were right on track, having already accumulated over a hundred miles. They lost some momentum a couple of months later when Robin broke a toe, but she recovered quickly and when we met again at the National Speakers Association convention in July, they were just ten miles behind schedule. By December 31, they had compiled 1,001 miles. They felt great, their clothes fit more loosely and they still knew the names of their offspring.

Demonstrating that exercise breeds discipline, Robin also managed to finish her first book that year.

Be Prepared

Wherever you go, if there is even a remote chance you could squeeze in a walk or some other workout, take along the appropriate gear. Pack shoes, shorts, sweats, hat, sunscreen, water bottle and whatever else you might need for those impromptu workout sessions.

On several occasions, I led morning walks at annual conventions and conferences of the National Speakers Association. Conference attendees often said to me in the elevators and the hallways, "I really want to join you on the walk, but I forgot my shoes."

Plan to Move on the Road

The key to staying reasonably fit in any time zone is to plan ahead. You may not match your regular exercise routine when you travel, but if you can schedule a few workouts, you won't have to start over again with your fit-

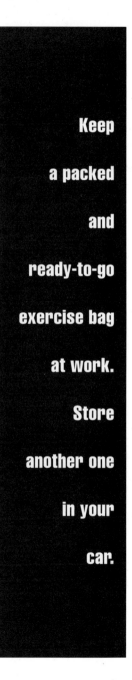

Keep a packed and ready-to-go exercise bag at work. Store another one in your car.

ness program when you get home. Before you leave the house, consider the following strategies.

• Call the visitor's bureau in your destination city. Ask about recreational activities you can enjoy during your stay. Gather information on hiking trails, bicycle routes and rentals, water sports, workout gyms and adventure companies.

• Request an aisle seat on your flight. You have more room in an aisle seat for stretching your arms above your head. When the pilot turns off the seatbelt sign, you can easily get out of an aisle seat to walk the cabin.

• Reserve a hotel with fitness facilities. You will save the time, hassle and expense of visiting a separate fitness facility — and you'll be more likely to use a gym that's conveniently located down the hall.

• Pack workout gear. Make room for walking shoes, workout clothes, workout tapes (and tape recorder) and an elastic band for toning or a strap for stretching.

A professional speaker told me that, although he loves the benefits of exercising while he is away on business, by the time he stuffs all his books and tapes into his suitcases, there is usually no room for his walking shoes.

If he truly appreciates what he gains from exercising on the road, he will pack his walking shoes first. If he arrives at his presentation with fewer books and tapes to sell, it won't hurt him in the long run.

By exercising regularly, he can sustain the strength and stamina to speak and sell his products for many more years.

• **Travel in shoes designed for walking.** You will be more inclined to cover some extra distance on foot during your travels. Your feet will thank you at the end of the day — and your heart and lungs will thank you, too.

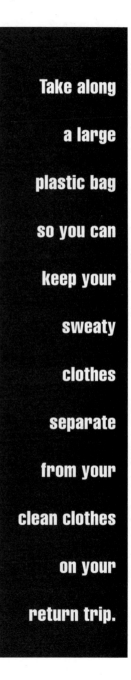

Take along a large plastic bag so you can keep your sweaty clothes separate from your clean clothes on your return trip.

Buy a daypack. It centers the load on your back and frees your hands. Get one with a waist strap, so some of the pack's weight shifts to your waist and lightens the load on your shoulders.

Move at the Airport

• **Explore the airport on foot.** After you check your heavy luggage, take a walk. Avoid conveyor belt walkways, or keep moving when you are on them.

• **Stretch.** Stretching relieves tension and helps prepare you mentally and physically for the flight ahead.

✔ Hold onto the back of a chair in the waiting area and step your right foot back about two feet.

✔ If you are wearing shoes with heels, remove them.

✔ Gently lower your right heel to the floor and slowly shift your hips forward. Feel a stretch in the back of your lower right leg.

✔ Breathe slowly and deeply as you hold the stretch for ten to twenty seconds, or as long as it feels comfortable.

✔ Release and repeat with the left leg.

If you notice people staring at you while you stretch, don't worry about it. Plenty of characters far stranger than you already hang out at airports.

Move on the Plane

• **Create your exercise itinerary.** When the pilot announces the plane has reached its cruising altitude, it's high time to crack open your planner, get out a red pen and block out specific times for physical activity during your days on the road. Do it now, before your mind and your agenda fill up with other matters.

• **As soon as the seat belt sign is turned off, move about the cabin.** Sitting for long periods in a cramped space can be brutal on the body, so roam the aisle and give your legs and back some relief. You might meet someone and make a business or personal connection. If you are having a great time working the crowd, ask the flight attendants if they need help passing out drinks.

• **Stand and stretch.** Stretch at your seat or, if the flight isn't full, move to the back of the cabin where you will have more room and be less inhibited.

✔ Slowly clasp your hands above your head. With your knees soft and your abdominal muscles pulled in, lift the left side of your ribcage toward the ceiling.

✔ Breathe. Feel a wonderful stretch along the left side of your body.

✔ Release and repeat on the other side.

If people near you begin to get nervous, describe how good it feels and invite them to join in. If you are feeling frisky, step to the front of the plane, turn and face the passengers and lead everyone through some stretches.

Move at Your Hotel

• **When you check in, check out the fitness facility.** On the way to your room, stop by the gym and sneak a peek. Notice the hours of operation and the gym's amenities. Are there aerobic stations such as treadmills or stationary bicycles? Are there weight machines? Are personal trainers available? Is there plenty of space and equipment, or should you plan to return during non-peak hours? The more you know about the gym, the more likely you are to make an appearance later — in your workout gear.

• **Work out in your hotel room.** Follow an exercise routine on TV, use audio or video tapes that you brought from home, or do your own aerobic, strength or stretch routine. If your workout involves some bouncy steps, be sure no one bigger than you is staying in the room below.

• **Take a walk from the hotel.** Ask the concierge for maps of recommended walking routes. Whenever possible, walk with someone and restrict your walks to daylight hours — unless the area is extremely well lit, crowded with people and obviously safe. If you do stray into an undesirable part of town, at least you will be inclined to move at a brisk pace.

• **Plan post-meal walks.** Not an arm-pumping, heart-pounding sprint, but a relaxing, stretch-your-legs saunter. Anticipating an after-meal stroll, you will be less likely to overeat. When your server asks what you would like for dessert, say "I'll take a walk, thank you."

When my friend Jack quit smoking, he filled the void with the much healthier habit of post-meal walking. Once or twice a day, Jack walks immediately after eating. In the process, he snuffed out his after-meal cigarette ritual. Thanks to these walks, Jack is slimmer today than when he was a smoker.

Move at Conventions/Conferences

• **Instead of a coffee break, take a "walkee" break.** If you have ten minutes, set your watch alarm for five minutes and start walking. If weather permits, step outside for a change of scenery. When your alarm beeps, turn around and retrace your steps. You will rejoin the meeting alert and refreshed.

• **Walk to a distant restroom.** This may be the best idea in this book. When the general session lets out and a flood of people streams out of the ballroom, you can avoid the long lines at the nearest restrooms by strolling down the hallway, striding around the corner and sauntering down the next hallway to another bathroom. At the remote restroom, you won't have to wait in line, and you will have squeezed some walking into your bathroom break.

Move During Non-Business Travel

We learn more about a person through an hour of play or games than a year of conversation.

—Plato

• **Announce your healthy intentions ahead of time.** Advise your relatives or friends of your plans to work out during your visit. They will

Request that exercise be added to next year's conference agenda. Scheduled sessions of walking, aerobics or yoga can raise the mood and energy level of participants and provide attendees with additional networking opportunities.

When possible, plan to exercise just before you were planning to shower anyway. You will save time — and water.

be more understanding of your needs, and they may even join you.

• **Organize physically active outings for family or friends.** Plan a walk in a forest or along a stream or at the seashore. Schedule an afternoon of horseback riding. Visit a park for a stroll or a few games of volleyball or badminton. Coordinate a leisurely bicycle ride. Besides benefiting everyone's health, group exercise encourages talking, sharing and laughter.

Plan Your Holiday Moves

Deborah, a former personal training client, once announced in mid-October that she wanted to take a break from her exercise sessions with me because the holidays were approaching and she would be too busy and too stressed to work out. After all, Halloween was only two weeks away, Thanksgiving was just around the corner and then there was Christmas.

Exercise is not a seasonal sport. Yet many people let their fitness routines lapse in late November and throughout the month of December, while stuffing their faces with holiday goodies. Then they rush to health clubs and spas in January to repair the damage they have done. It doesn't have to be this way. With a little healthy planning, you can keep moving — and stay fit — twelve months a year.

First, plan an attitude shift from: *"Gosh, I'm so busy this time of year, I don't have time for my fitness,"* to: *"During this stressful time of year, I need my exercise more than ever."*

Second, use the following strategies:

• **Pre-pay your December workouts.** Feeling a financial commitment, you may get to the gym more often.

• **Schedule something special during December.**

✔ Take ice skating or cross country ski lessons.

✔ Begin a stationary bike ride across your state.

✔ Take an active vacation. Early December is a quiet, no-hassle travel period and a timely occasion to recharge your batteries. You will return home ready to continue your healthy rejuvenation into the new year.

• **Strengthen your support system.** Invite a friend to join you for a 10K charity walk in early December.

If you exercise with friends and some members of the group are feeling crazed from the pressures of the season, that's all the more reason to meet in December. You all need the escape. If necessary, shift a date or two to accommodate everyone's schedule, but do not skip your December exercise sessions entirely. They are likely to be the most necessary — and the most appreciated — workouts of the year.

• **Plan a healthy holiday party.** Focus on fitness and fun, not food. If there's snow on the ground, meet friends and family for ice skating at a local rink, downhill skiing at a nearby ski resort or cross country skiing in a convenient park. If the weather is decent, set up a net for volleyball or badminton or walk to the park and fly kites. Organize a group hike or a walk or bike ride through your neighborhood. If the weather stinks, take your party indoors for ping pong, hire a professional to give dance lessons at your house or invite your friends to climb the walls — literally — at an indoor climbing gym.

Your active event should be a big hit. Instead of feeling post-party guilt and lethargy from their millionth holiday eat-and-drink-athon, your guests will leave invigorated and thankful.

• **Practice healthy gift-giving.** Gift certificates for exercise equipment, clothes and footwear, massages, yoga classes, a day spa, a short-term or introductory membership in a health club — all make thoughtful gifts. Drop strong hints to all your friends and relatives that you would love to receive fitness-related presents.

If one advances confidently in the direction of his

dreams, and endeavors to lead the life which he

has imagined, he will meet with a success

unexpected in common hours.

—Henry David Thoreau

Your Ten-Minute Solution™

Before you turn the page, complete the following:

✔ **Schedule ten minutes of exercise every other day this week.** Highlight the exact days and times on your calendar — in red ink.

✔ **Create a healthy travel checklist.** File it with papers connected with your next trip. When you start packing, you will see your list of fitness items to take along. Let me get you started:

❏ Walking shoes   ❏ Audio/video exercise tapes

❏ Workout clothes ❏ Tape recorder and batteries

✔ **List three non-exercise activities you enjoy.** If you like to go to the movies, the library or visit friends, choose a reasonable destination and schedule a walk or bike ride in the next week.

Step 4:
Gather Support

One of the best ways you can bolster your resolve to become fit and stay fit is to surround yourself with fit-minded friends. If you wish to live a healthier lifestyle, spend more time with your non-smoking, healthy-eating and physically-active comrades. They will encourage you to stick with the good habits you already have, and they may inspire you to drop a few more of your bad habits.

Other ways you can gather support for your new lifestyle include:

• **Recruit a workout partner or two.** You can't always do it alone. Sometimes you can develop more consistency with your fitness if someone else is depending on you.

Suppose you plan to walk at daybreak on Saturday, but when your alarm jolts you awake at 7:00 a.m. you decide an early morning workout on the weekend is a dumb idea. Just before you roll over and return to dreamland, you remember that you promised to meet a friend at a local park in twenty minutes. Guilt works. You leap out of bed, slip on your workout gear and head out the door.

• **Embrace diversity.** Openly discuss with your workout companion that the two of you may have different needs or abilities. With some compromise, each of you should enjoy the workout you deserve.

When I hike with Sandy, we walk together on the level and downhill sections of trail while we discuss what is new in our lives and attempt to solve the pressing problems in the world. As we begin the long uphill climb, I usually go ahead at a faster pace and spend a minute or two at the top of the hill stretching until Sandy catches up. We each get the workout we want, and we get plenty of time to socialize, too.

If that doesn't work for you, look for several workout partners, some at your level of fitness, some who will challenge you. Then alternate days and activities.

• **Join a gym.** The facility, with its set schedule of classes, can provide the structure you need to complete workouts you would not have the discipline to schedule and do on your own at home. Better yet, join a gym with a friend. That way, you have the added support of a workout partner.

• **Join a walking, hiking or bicycling club.** The social interaction makes each workout fun and motivating. Be sure to read the event descriptions in the club newsletter carefully so you pick outings that match your abilities and interests. Then just show up at the scheduled time and follow the leader.

• **Seek support in your community.** Register for a walk, ride or other fitness event. As you visualize the up-

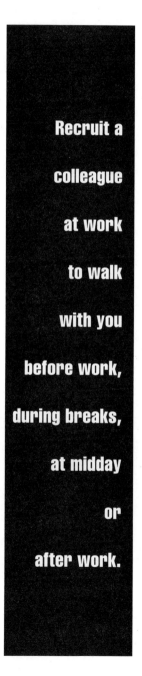

Recruit a colleague at work to walk with you before work, during breaks, at midday or after work.

> **Pay ahead for a block of ten exercise classes and you are more likely to attend class regularly, especially if those ten sessions must be completed by a certain date.**

coming event, with you moving among hundreds of fellow exercise enthusiasts, you will be eager to get in shape for the big day.

• **Form a Hike-A-Month club.** Your mission statement can be: *to maintain an active membership with special people in spectacular locations.*

Take these steps:

✔ Invite two or more friends to become charter members of your club.

✔ Agree on a day of the month to meet (perhaps every third Saturday).

✔ Purchase a book on hiking trails in your area.

✔ From the trails book, select a hike for your first gathering.

Consider the fitness level of your friends. If you start with a super strenuous hike, they may not be your friends for long.

✔ Meet at the trailhead (carpool, if possible).

✔ After your hike, hand the book to another club member, who will choose next month's excursion.

When I lived in Northern California, I was a charter member of a hike-a-month club with two close friends. Sometimes other friends tagged along on our hikes, and occasionally we revised our meeting date to accommodate our various schedules. Nevertheless, for two-and-a-half years, we explored the open space of

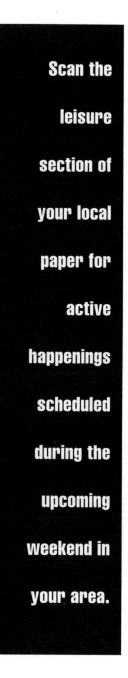

Scan the leisure section of your local paper for active happenings scheduled during the upcoming weekend in your area.

> If bad weather prevents your hike or bike group from operating year round, form a cross country ski or ice skate-a-month club. Or venture indoors for aerobics, dance, circuit training or yoga.

the San Francisco Bay Area, and we never missed a month.

We did not stay fit by hiking once a month, but we did stay fit thanks to our hike-a-month club. None of us wanted to be the weak link that would slow down the group, so each of us was highly motivated to stay in reasonable shape between meetings.

We were amazed by the variety and number of scenic trails just a short drive from civilization. Check out the wilderness areas near you, gather up the people you would like to share special moments with, and go explore the wilds. You, too, may discover that hours spent with friends in a natural setting is time well spent.

• **Combine exercise with other matters.** If you can accomplish two things at once, you're more likely to find the time to work out. While you are hiking, walking, running, stretching, using a stair machine or pedaling a stationary bicycle, you can listen to tapes on professional or personal growth topics or enjoy your favorite music. Indoors, you can exercise while you catch up on television news or your favorite soap opera.

While you're hiking or walking, you can listen to a taped rehearsal of a presentation you will be giving soon, or actually rehearse your speech. The physical movement will energize your rehearsal and help transfer that energy to your upcoming presentation.

People in creative jobs often find that detaching themselves from the workplace and going for a brisk walk will help ideas to jell. New approaches or concepts will often strike like lightning, in a synergistic response to exercise. Carry a small notebook or pad and pencil with you.

• **Go Netwalking**™. If you need to network or brainstorm one-on-one with a client or colleague, replace the traditional sit-down meeting over bacon and eggs with a healthier alternative: **Netwalking**™...*where business matters are discussed afoot.*

Netwalking™ can improve the health of your relationships in more ways than one. The outdoor environment, far from the chaos of a crowded and noisy restaurant, can create a relaxed atmosphere for the two of you. The physical movement, besides being healthy for your bodies, can stimulate creative thinking. Walking side by side, you and your **Netwalking**™ partner can feel equal in status.

• **Be a source of support.** Set a healthy example with your active lifestyle, and your family and friends may follow your lead. It's a win/win strategy.

Your desire to cast a healthy influence on other people will strengthen your own exercise program.

Consider a Personal Fitness Trainer

You might benefit from the support of one-on-one attention. Not everyone needs, wants or can afford a personal trainer but, for some people, a trainer can be the answer to sagging motivation or problems fitting exercise into a hectic schedule. You could benefit from a personal trainer if you need extra motivation to work out on your own (even after reading this book), you need instruction on the proper use of your home exercise equipment or you need instruction on the equipment at your gym.

When looking for a personal trainer, decide whether you wish to be trained in your home or at a gym. Then ask friends and acquaintances for referrals to competent trainers. If your friends can't help, ask the staff at local fitness facilities for referrals.

Ask prospective trainers about their experience, their qualifications, degrees, certifications and professional affiliations and their areas of expertise — aerobics, strength training,

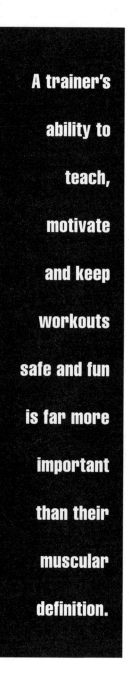

A trainer's ability to teach, motivate and keep workouts safe and fun is far more important than their muscular definition.

stretching, yoga, nutrition, etc. Then ask how they can help you achieve your particular fitness goals. Make sure you have a clear understanding of what they charge and how payment must be made. Finally, get names of some of their current clients and permission to call some for feedback.

After you meet with a prospective trainer, ask yourself if you enjoyed their company. Did they listen to you? Did they ask about your interests and goals as well as details of your medical history (including medications, ailments and injuries)? Were they safety conscious? Spending the time and energy up front to find a trainer that suits your needs will pay off big time.

How often you meet with a trainer depends on your objectives. If you are looking for motivation, two or three sessions a week may be necessary. If you want to learn correct technique, meet two or three times a week initially, then once every week or two until your technique is consistently good.

Your Ten-Minute Solution™

Before you turn the page, complete the following:

✔ **Write down where you want to be with your exercise program six months from now.** Be as specific as possible. Seal your plan inside a self-addressed, stamped envelope, send it to a friend, and ask them to mail it back to you when that date arrives.

✔ **Jot down the names of three local friends you have been neglecting.** Call and invite one or all of them to join you on a walk for the purpose of catching up on each other's lives. Set a specific date and time.

✔ **Make a note on your calendar to check Thursday's paper for a listing of active happenings.** Then choose one to do.

Step 5:
Balance Your Workouts

When you have been exercising for one or two months, it's time to evaluate the kinds of exercise you're doing. Are you still doing just one thing, or have you started to mix it up, altering your workouts for variety and balance?

Balance your workouts and you are more likely to stick with exercise for the long term. With a well-rounded exercise program, you maximize your benefits, minimize your risk of injury and greatly reduce the chance that boredom will rear its ugly head. Your workouts will stay varied and interesting, and you will stay committed.

The best way to add balance is to include the three exercise essentials — aerobics, strength training and stretching — in your workouts each week. Each component offers unique advantages.

Aerobics

An aerobic workout burns fat, feels good and strengthens your heart/lung system. Since heart disease is the number one cause of death for men and women in America, keeping your heart strong is a mighty good idea.

Get aerobic by elevating your heart rate for a sustained period of at least fifteen to twenty minutes. You can walk, run, swim, bicycle, cross country ski, take an aerobics class or work on an aerobic machine at home or in a gym, or do any other activity that works many of the major muscle groups of the body and gets your heart pumping. Try to do an aerobic workout at least three or four days a week.

• **Monitor your intensity.** You do this with "Perceived Exertion" — which simply means paying attention to how you feel. On a scale from 0 to 10, rate the intensity of your workout. At 0 you are lying on a couch; at 5 you are exercising at a moderate level of intensity; at 10 you are collapsing from exhaustion. Shoot for 4 to 7 on the Perceived Exertion scale, and you will strengthen your cardiovascular system and burn fat—without placing undue stress on the heart.

Strength Training

*Resistance training is NOT
when a person refuses to be
trained.*

—JS

Strength training, also known as weight training or resistance training, speeds up your metabolism, builds and tones muscle and increases bone mass (especially important for women, who are at greater risk of developing osteoporosis).

Regular weight training enables you to perform everyday lifting, pushing, pulling and carrying chores with confidence and without injury.

• **Do at least ten minutes of strength exercises** (using machines or hand weights, or simply doing cal-

When you are exercising, always be able to pass the talk test. If you cannot talk, you are pushing too hard. If you can still sing, you may not be working hard enough.

> **Spend your resting time between sets stretching the muscle group you have just worked. That way, you make time for stretching without lengthening your workout.**

isthenics) on two or three non-con-secutive days each week. Your safety and success depends on proper technique, so consult with a fitness trainer if you need help with your form.

• **Focus on upper body exercises.** With the proliferation of treadmills, stationary bicycles and stair climbers, it's easy to target your lower body with your aerobic workouts. Your upper body probably needs attention.

• **Develop a simple *take-me-anywhere* strength routine.** When I travel, I work my upper body by doing three sets (twelve to fifteen repetitions per set) of push-ups and dips, then performing isolated contractions of my abdominal and back muscles. I can complete my *take-me-*

anywhere strength routine in ten to twelve minutes (not including my warm-up). This routine feels good and energizes me, and I can do it anywhere. The only equipment I need is a chair (for the dips).

• **Add push-ups to your routine.** The push-up is the single best upper body exercise. It strengthens the chest, shoulders, arms, back and wrists.

✔ Begin with the beginner push-up (on your knees with your hips bent at a ninety degree angle).

✔ When that's easy for you, graduate to the intermediate version (on your knees with your hips extended so you form a straight line from head to knees). Check your form in a full-length mirror.

✔ When you can perform the intermediate version easily, you can either do advanced push-ups (on toes with body straight from feet to head) or increase the number of repetitions. The intermediate push-up is adequate to develop a reasonable amount of strength.

Note: The purpose of this book is to get you moving, not to describe specific exercises. For appropriate exercises and instruction on proper form, see a fitness instructor or trainer.

Stretching

> *Stretching, like Rodney Dangerfield, gets no respect. When a fitness instructor asks you if you stretch, you usually respond the same as when your dentist asks you if you floss: "Well, yeah, but not as much as I should."*
>
> —JS

Stretching can increase flexibility, reduce muscle soreness, lower stress, decrease risk of injury, heal and prevent back problems, improve posture and enhance your golf or tennis game by increasing the range of motion of your swing.

Stretching also feels good.

Other than that, I can't think of any reason to stretch.

• **Stretch every day for at least five to ten minutes.** The best time is right after a workout, since warm muscles stretch more easily than cold ones.

✔ Hold each stretch for ten to twenty seconds, or as long as the stretch is comfortable.

✔ Be pain free. Move into a stretch slowly. If it hurts, back off a bit or release the stretch.

✔ Do not bounce. Jerky movements can tear muscles.

✔ Breathe slowly and deeply. Deep breathing is relaxing, and a relaxed muscle stretches more readily.

✔ See a trainer to learn specific stretches, or order my stretch audio tape (see form in the back of this book).

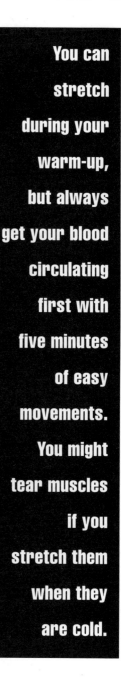

You can stretch during your warm-up, but always get your blood circulating first with five minutes of easy movements. You might tear muscles if you stretch them when they are cold.

Spend extra time stretching your tightest muscle group. If the hamstring muscles in back of your upper legs are tight, do a stretch for your hamstrings, then repeat the same stretch. With extra attention, they will begin to loosen up.

Always Warm Up and Cool Down

Make it a habit to start and finish with the bookends of a balanced workout. A five- or ten-minute warm-up period up front will help prevent injury and prepare your body for exercise.

Cooling down or slowing your pace gradually during the final five minutes of your workout will help prevent lightheadedness and dizziness.

Balance the Frequency of Your Workouts

Move your body in some way at least every other day. Better yet, after a month or two, increase to five or six days a week. While taking at least one day off each week is a good idea to help you remain physically and mentally refreshed, you could work out seven days a week and still keep your sanity and your safety — if those weekly workouts feature plenty of variety.

Work out too hard or too often, especially doing the same activity, and you risk injury or burnout.

Awhile ago, a friend called me and excitedly reported, "Joe, you'll be proud of me. My husband and I started an exercise program, and every morning I walk the treadmill while he rides the stationary bicycle. We work out for an hour and we've done it for nine days in a row!"

"Well... congratulations," I said cautiously, "but have you considered taking a day off once in awhile?"

She responded, "Are you allowed to do that?"

A few months later, we spoke again. She and her husband were no longer exercising.

Design a Time-Efficient Workout

After you move beyond the beginner level, you can fit the key components of exercise in one forty-five minute session.

The following workout, using walking as an example, includes aerobics, toning and stretching, as well as the mandatory warm-up and cool-down.

10 minutes	walk slowly	warm-up phase
20 minutes	walk faster	aerobic and toning phase
5 minutes	walk slowly	cool-down phase
10 minutes	stretch	stretch phase

45 minutes TOTAL

• **Work your weaknesses.** Devote extra time to your problem areas and they will improve. As Bob Peavy, one of my gymnastics coaches, used to say, "Everything gets easier with practice."

If you lack upper body strength, work your upper body at least two days a week and you will get stronger.

If you have trouble touching your toes, take a yoga class at least twice a week and you will loosen up considerably.

If you have a tough time climbing hills, climb more hills, and eventually they will get easier. If you lack coordination, take an aerobics or dance class or sign up for volleyball.

You can develop some athletic ability, if you are willing to face your weaknesses head-on.

• **Do activities that balance your lifestyle.** If you are a librarian, a loud, high-energy aerobics class may be just what you need. If you are a stockbroker, you already get enough noise and excitement in your life. Seek peace with tai chi, stretching or yoga.

• **Try yoga.** Yoga is a discipline with *balance* written all over it. Yoga can improve your posture and flexibility, and many forms of yoga build strength as well. The deep breathing exercises in yoga can help you release tension that you may have been carrying around for years.

Ashtanga Yoga can even get your heart pumping with a flowing series

Keep your expectations in balance by accepting your basic body shape. Shooting for model-thin or Hulk Hogan-big is unrealistic, stressful and unhealthy. Strive to become a more vibrant version of your present self.

> Yoga styles and teachers can vary tremendously, so if your first session is not what you hoped for, visit another studio until you find a style of yoga your body and your mind respond to.

of postures that strengthens and stretches your muscles.

It has only taken a few thousand years, but the fitness community is finally embracing yoga as a legitimate form of exercise.

Jill, the wife of my best friend, suffered with sciatica (inflammation of the sciatic nerve) in her mid-thirties. She experienced discomfort in the buttocks and pain shooting down both legs all the way to her feet. At her doctor's recommendation, she was spending most of every day in bed, with two or three brief breaks daily to shuffle carefully to the bathroom. Formerly cheerful and energetic, Jill became deeply depressed and exhibited the physical traits of a slow-moving centenarian.

I mentioned to Jill that some yoga stretches might bring her some relief, and I offered to show her a few poses. She shuddered at the thought of moving her body, but I assured her that we would proceed slowly and cautiously so no position would aggravate her condition. She nervously allowed me to guide her through a few seated and lying poses on the carpet in their living room.

To her surprise — and my relief — she enjoyed the exercises and actually felt better by the end of our brief session. For several days thereafter, we repeated the yoga postures and stretches. Delighted with the results, Jill enrolled in a yoga class in her town.

A few months later, Jill reported she was progressing well with her yoga classes, and she was spending more time in motion and less time in pain.

I never met a yoga class I didn't like.

—JS

• **Try something new.** More exercise variations are available today than ever before. Many of them have strange sounding names, but just because you can't pronounce it or spell it doesn't mean you shouldn't try it. Consider pilates, feldenkreis, tai chi and other "new" exercises (many have actually been around for a long time). Find out if they'll work for you.

Keep an open mind and you may be pleasantly surprised. You might discover a style of exercise that fits you like a glove, one that adds the balance your exercise has needed all along.

Your Ten-Minute Solution™

Before you turn the page, complete the following:

✔ **Identify the weakest element or missing component of your exercise program** (aerobics, strength training, stretching or a proper warm-up or cool-down).

✔ **Schedule at least two ten-minute sessions this week to work specifically on your weakness.**

✔ **Do one of those ten-minute sessions right now.** If your posture is poor, concentrate on the posture string for the next ten minutes. If you need stretching, walk for five minutes as a warm-up, then stretch the areas of your body that need it the most.

Step 6:
Take Active Vacations

Vacation (va-ka' shen) n. A period of time
devoted to pleasure, rest or relaxation.

American Heritage Dictionary

Did you return home from your last vacation in need of a vacation to recover from your vacation? Were you feeling fat, sluggish, stressed and out of shape? Maybe you spent your days stuck to car seats, sequestered on tour buses or glued to a lounge chair, and your only opportunity for exercise was lugging your suitcase through the airport or adjusting the rearview mirror on your car. If that scenario sounds familiar, you could benefit from a more *moving* experience.

An active vacation is the closest thing to a quick fix. In only one week, you can turn around a bad attitude about fitness — and get started on developing good health habits at the same time. If you are already physically fit, an active vacation can strengthen your commitment to your active lifestyle.

Appreciate the Advantages

You can gain more

from a one-week active vacation than from

ten years of reading articles on health.

—JS

An active vacation will actually help you relax and de-stress better than a sedentary vacation. And it gives you an excuse not to visit Great-Aunt Martha's farm *again*. Other benefits include:

• **You can eat without guilt.** Knowing you will have plenty of calorie-burning opportunities on your trip, you can re-fuel at every meal without hesitation or trepidation.

• **You get motivated.** You are inspired to get in shape ahead of time so you will enjoy the trip more and get your money's worth. During your vacation, you find it incredibly easy to make time for exercise, since physical activity is the central theme and everyone around you is active. When you return home, possibly in the best shape of your life, you are eager to keep moving so you can maintain your new level of fitness.

• **You can escape.** Whether you are maneuvering a raft through rapids and around house-sized boulders, or you are coasting down a tree-lined country road on a mountain bike at dusk when two deer suddenly dart across your path fifty feet in front of you, you will find it very easy to forget your everyday problems.

• **You can have a ton of fun.** A fitness resort often resembles a camp for adults, offering playful activities such as water volleyball, tennis, dancing, hiking, improvisational comedy games and bingo. Pace yourself. Your smile muscles may be in for a vigorous workout.

• **You can raise your self-worth.** By completing a

physical challenge — whether it is seven days of classes at a spa, miles of whitewater rapids in a kayak or a week's worth of touring by bicycle — you can boost your confidence and self-esteem significantly because of your accomplishments.

• **You can lock onto memories that will last for a lifetime** — and inspire others to do the same.

A few years ago, while I was hiking with a local outdoor club, a woman in our group started talking about her ten-day rafting trip down the Colorado River through the Grand Canyon. As we hiked for the next hour, she described her whitewater venture with such vivid detail and enthusiasm, I assumed she had only recently returned from her vacation. Actually, her adventure had occurred two years earlier!

Thanks to that woman, I gave new attention to my long-time dream of rafting the same route. A year later, I completed my journey floating down the Colorado River through the Grand Canyon.

• **You can change your life.** When you are immersed in a program of physical activity for several days, surrounded by people with similar goals, the impact can be powerful and permanent. When you return home from an active vacation, you may decide once and for all to turn your attitude completely around and commit to a healthy lifestyle for life.

Brent is a case in point. His life was out of control. He earned an excellent income as a doctor, but he also worked long hours, smoked three packs of cigarettes a day and suffered from ulcers. His visit to a fitness resort redirected his life.

During his week at the spa, Brent realized that dying prematurely from his unhealthy habits and leaving his wife financially secure might be responsible, but it was certainly foolish. He decided he would rather make less money and be around longer to help his wife spend it.

When Brent returned home, he trimmed his medical practice and expanded his active vacation practice. During the next few years, he and his wife enjoyed treks, bicycle tours and even a week on horseback herding cattle with real cowboys.

They also continued their annual visit to the spa that turned Brent's life around.

Consider Your Options

• **Travel by bicycle.** Imagine you're on a bicycle tour in Vermont during the peak of the fall foliage season. Pedaling at your own pace, you stop whenever the urge strikes — to chat with the local folks, to browse the quaint shops in the small villages or to capture on film the brilliant oranges, yellows and reds that blanket the hillsides. At midday, a congenial group of co-travelers convenes at a scenic spot where your leaders prepare and serve a tasty and generous picnic-style lunch.

If rain threatens to dampen your day or you grow tired of pedaling, you flag down the support van, which will transport you to this evening's accommodation, a charming nineteenth century country inn. At the end of the day, after soothing your sore muscles in the Jacuzzi, you enjoy a hearty five-course meal with the group, while laughter and stories of the day's experiences bounce around the table. You discover that camaraderie spreads fast among people sharing the same adventure.

The next morning, while feasting on a breakfast of whole-grain pancakes and locally-produced maple syrup, you notice your tour leaders are outside tuning the bikes, wiping road dust off the frames and pumping air into the tires. For a moment, you feel a twinge of guilt, but it soon passes. Hey, it's not your job to do the dirty work — you're on vacation!

• **Travel by trekking.** From gentle walking excursions to high-altitude mountain treks, tour companies can lead you to exotic destinations around the globe.

Our home base for a six-day hiking tour in the Lake District of England was a 200-year-old farmhouse on a working farm. Each morning, a van shuttled us to a different trailhead. The hiking was splendid, with plenty of variety, gorgeous scenery, and the support and encouragement of guides and co-travelers. Some days included literary workouts as well, featuring visits — on foot — to Wordsworth's and Beatrix Potter's homes.

The food was phenomenal. Two young local women cooked our meals and prepared sandwiches and snacks for us to carry on our outings. Each day, when we returned from our hike, we were greeted by the aroma of baked breads the moment we entered the house. Even after a grueling all-day hike, I didn't care if someone beat me to the shower. I patiently waited my turn by the fireplace, sipping hot tea and devouring warm, moist muffins fresh out of the oven.

Our hike leaders split our group into three subgroups. The fittest individuals hiked the most challenging trails and, by the end of the week, they had scaled the three highest peaks in England.

The moderately-fit group trekked rolling hills, avoiding steep slopes and long ascents. Two individuals who were not fit enough to hike were shuttled each day to a different village where they could spend the day strolling, frequenting the shops and enjoying the sights.

Each day began and concluded with a session of stretching or yoga. The morning class woke us up and prepared our bodies for hiking. The early evening session lengthened our muscles and reduced soreness. We enjoyed the stretching as much as the muffins and afternoon tea.

• **Travel on skis.** Besides hiking and biking, you can

cross-country ski from inn to inn. In New England, for instance, you can stay in a Victorian manor one evening and on a sprawling country estate the next night. Your active vacation need not be limited to the warm months.

• **Visit a dude ranch.** Life on a ranch can be wonderfully varied. You might return to the days of the Wild West and drive cattle by horseback across miles of sagebrush, camping under the stars with real wranglers.

Then again, your ranch vacation may feature tennis, swimming, whitewater rafting, fishing and massage. Look forward to home-cooked meals, old-fashioned hospitality and a simpler and slower pace.

• **Visit a fitness resort.** Immerse yourself in a week devoted to your health. Participate in a wide range of exercise classes, discover numerous techniques for managing stress, and enjoy three nutritious, low-fat, high-energy meals a day.

Some spas pamper you, providing a personal trainer, your own schedule and daily treatments ranging from massages to herbal wraps and from facials to pedicures. Other resorts offer a smorgasbord of physical activities. You pick and choose from the extensive fitness menu and determine how active your week will be.

This could be a typical day at a spa:

6:30 a.m.-7:30 a.m.
Begin the day with an invigorating hike.

8 a.m.-9 a.m.
Fuel your body with whole grain cereals, freshly baked breads and an abundant selection of fresh fruit.

9 a.m., 10 a.m. & 11 a.m.
Choose from yoga, stretching, toning, weight training, aerobics, dance, pool exercises, volleyball, tennis, fitness walking, back care and more. Most classes are forty-five minutes in length.

12 noon-1:30 p.m.
Make your selections from the lunch buffet: vegetables, pastas, casseroles, soups and breads.

2 p.m., 3 p.m. & 4 p.m.
More exercise options, just like in the morning. The four o'clock hour emphasizes relaxation.

5 p.m.
Lectures and workshops in nutrition, stress management, meditation or jewelry making.

6 p.m.-7:30 p.m.
Dinner is served in the dining room as you and fellow spa guests recap the events of the day and plan for new ones.

8 p.m.

Although fitness resorts are not known for their night life, you could:

- watch a movie
- attend an evening lecture that entertains, informs or inspires
- socialize or play cards or a board game in the lounge
- return to your room to catch up on your reading
- return to your room, put your head on your pillow and start dreaming of tomorrow's bowl of oatmeal.

I haven't had any alcohol,

cigarettes or salt for a week

— and I don't miss them.

—a spa guest

- **Whet your appetite with a water adventure.** Sign up for a rafting, kayaking or canoeing trip, or pick a package tour that features snorkeling,

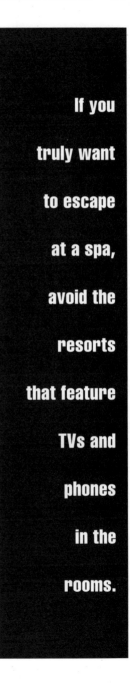

If you

truly want

to escape

at a spa,

avoid the

resorts

that feature

TVs and

phones

in the

rooms.

Designate a drawer for information on active vacations. Having a place to keep all those colorful brochures will help you select the right adventure later.

board sailing and other water activities all at one location.

Imagine a week without using your credit card, telephone or car keys; without seeing a newspaper, television or billboard; without hearing a radio, an obnoxious leaf-blower or car alarm; without worrying about preparing your next meal. That's what I experienced on my rafting adventure down the Colorado River through the Grand Canyon.

Each morning, big-horn sheep and white-tailed deer served as nature's billboards, standing along the riverbank as we silently floated by. The canyon wren's melodic whistle greeted us each day from the shoreline, replacing civilization's constant drone from radios, cars and jet planes.

Each day featured stretches of calming, peaceful water, interspersed with white-knuckle rapids that put us on the edge of our seats and nearly tossed us out of them. At least twice a day we parked our rafts on shore and explored caves, searched for fossils, hiked through narrow side canyons to spring-fed waterfalls and swimming holes, or visited 1,000-year-old Indian ruins.

During the calm sections of river, our trip leader told fascinating stories, relating the history of the region and showcasing the early explorers of the area. I learned about John Wesley Powell who, in 1869, despite having only one arm, bravely led the first boat expedition through the Grand Canyon.

To our constant relief, the crew skillfully maneuvered the rafts through swift-moving whitewater and around huge boulders. Yet their greatest performance may have been meal preparation. When our boats glided onto a sandy beach for a lunch break, they leapt onto shore and proceeded to set up tables, slice tomatoes, onions and avocados, break apart heads of lettuce, unload cheese, luncheon meats and loaves of bread and set out condiments and snacks. Within minutes, the sandwich-making buffet line was in operation.

Breakfast and dinner were no less impressive. The morning menu featured omelets served to order, French toast, blueberry pancakes, waffles or oatmeal. Cereal, toast and fruit were available every morning. The evening meal always included salad, vegetables and dessert, while the main course might be barbecued chicken, fish, lasagna, spaghetti or pork chops.

The thirty people in our group (two boats, fifteen to a craft), discovered that when strangers share an adventure, friendships develop quite easily. These river enthusiasts came from all corners of the U.S. and represented a variety of professions. After mixing with the group for a few days, I realized I was in good company. I theorized that if a rock broke loose from the canyon wall and struck me, Joel (the nurse) could administer first aid; if the rock were to hit me in the jaw, Dan (the ear, nose and throat doctor) could diagnose my condition; if I decided to take legal action, Pam (the personal injury attorney) could represent me; and if I were just curious, Pete (the geologist) could tell me the age of the rock that hit me.

• **Plan an environmental vacation.** With over 100 different projects available each year around the globe, there's a subject to satisfy everyone's tastes. Most expeditions are physically active. Working beside a scientist, you can study Rocky Mountain wildflowers in Colorado, analyze volcanoes in Costa Rica, teach dolphins a language in Hawaii or dig up dinosaur bones in Montana. You may not think of the excavation of an archaeological site as a vacation, but it could be the best vacation of all — a total departure from your regular routine.

In 1989, I spent twelve days as a member of a research team tracking mountain lions in the Idaho wilderness. We were studying the impact of fragmented habitat on the welfare of the North American lion. Using radio telemetry equipment, we monitored the movements of two collared cats, Butch and Lola, and we gained knowledge and insight about these elusive animals that could never have been gathered from books.

We also garnered much satisfaction from contributing not just money, but brain, muscle and sweat to what we considered a worthwhile cause. The hiking we did in the Sawtooth Mountains was substantial, and our working environment was spectacular.

- **Get active with a special interest group.** Many spas or tour outfits cater to special populations. They offer exclusive weeks for women, men, singles, couples, families or seniors. Some hiking tours cater to bird-watchers or photographers. Sign up your family for a bicycle tour during "family" week and one child may ride for free.

Corporations are discovering healthy alternatives to traditional getaways. Appreciating the team-building, morale-boosting and stress-releasing potential of active vacations, companies are sending executives, managers and staff on bicycle tours, rafting trips, sailing camps and fitness resorts for unique, healthy retreats.

Check Your Sources

More active vacation choices are available today than ever

before — and plenty of information is out there. On the Internet, you can type in keywords "active vacations" and go from there.

However, if you're already too sedentary, keep your Internet time brief. Don't let technology rob you of your fitness. Balance your on-line time with your "on feet" time.

• **Let your fingers do the walking.** Visit the back pages of bicycling, walking, backpacking, nature, outdoor photography, multisport, water sport, travel and spa magazines for toll-free numbers of adventure companies and spas. Request brochures and catalogs for the tour events that catch your eye. To get you started, see the resource list in the appendix at the back of this book.

• **Contact your travel agent.** Increasing numbers of travel agencies work with active vacations and spa holidays. Some agents actually take groups to fitness resorts every year and are intimately familiar with the spa experience.

• **Ask your local fitness professionals.** Fitness instructors and personal trainers at your health club may have a personal connection with active vacations. Some of them may have worked for a tour company or at a fitness resort, and other fitness staff probably have worked with clients who have vacationed at a fitness resort.

• **Ask your friends.** You probably know someone who has enjoyed an active vacation. They will be delighted to share details of their adventure with you. They may even invite you to their house to view a few carousels of slides or a videotape or ten.

You have been warned.

Pick the Right Trip for You

Read the small print in the trip brochure. Be sure you understand:

✔ the recommended fitness level

✔ the size of the group

✔ the type, quality and quantity of food served

✔ possible weather conditions

✔ how much free time is scheduled

✔ what a typical day is like

✔ the type of accommodations.

When in doubt, choose a fitness resort. If you have no idea what physical activities you might enjoy for a week because you rarely move your body, then visit a spa. With dozens of activities to choose from, if you don't find an exercise that moves you, at least you'll enjoy the massages, the meals and the relaxing environment.

Get In Shape Before Your Vacation

Smart people take active
vacations to shape up.
Brilliant people shape up,
then take active vacations.

—JS

Arrive fit and you can participate in most activities without fear of injury, exhaustion or sore muscles. Arrive fit

Pack the right gear. Read the "items to bring" list carefully, highlighting the things that apply to your vacation. Read it again when you think you have finished packing.

and you'll enjoy and get the most out of your active vacation. Here's how to get in shape:

• **Start early.** Get active four weeks to three months ahead of time. The more physically challenging your vacation will be, the more time you need to prepare. Put down a deposit as early as possible, because the moment you read your credit card number over the phone, you will feel an urge to get moving.

• **Train specifically.** Any physical activity will help, but sport-specific activities work best. To train for a bicycle tour, get on your bike. If you are signed up for a hilly walking tour, take hikes on hilly terrain or raise the slope during your treadmill practice.

• **Build gradually.** If you're not already active, start with the **10-15-20 Approach**™ (see Step 2). Every month, add another workout to your week until you are exercising five or six days a week.

Waiting till the last week to shape up is foolish. Too often, I have met people at the resort who arrived injured because they crammed in too much exercise just before going on vacation. They were not happy campers. They spent much of their frustrating week watching all the healthy guests cheerfully partake in the activities.

Take Your Vacation Home With You

Your active week is special. Yet the greatest benefit of an active vacation may be the lingering effect for months, years or a lifetime. Here's how to make sure your active vacation doesn't end the moment you return home:

• **Plan ahead.** Arrive knowing what you want to get out of your week. If you hope to lift weights regularly at your local gym when you return home, be sure to attend the strength training classes at the spa.

• **Schedule at least two active events a year.** Many spa guests tell me that they take new habits home for about six months, then they fall apart. To prevent this from happening to you, plan two active getaways a year, six months apart. Just when you are losing the residuals from your most recent trip, you'll start getting psyched up for your next active holiday. If budget and time restraints limit you to one week-long vacation per year, then set aside a long week-end for your second adventure. Your mini-adventure could be a three-day backpacking trip, a rafting trip, a bicycle tour or a rock-climbing weekend.

Twenty years from now,

you will be more disappointed

by the things you didn't do

than by the ones you did do.

So throw off the bowlines.

Sail away from the safe harbor.

Catch the trade winds in your sails.

Explore.

Dream.

Discover.

—Mark Twain

Your Ten-Minute Solution™

Before you turn the page, complete the following:

✔ **Turn to the appendix and call at least three active vacation outfits.** Request their brochures and catalogues.

✔ **List three friends or acquaintances who have taken active vacations.** Call them and ask which trips and outfits or spas they recommend. Get the toll-free numbers of the outfits they like. Ask for the phone numbers of other people they know who have also taken active vacations.

✔ **Create a file for active vacation brochures.**

Step 7:
Make Exercise A Priority

If I had known I was going to live this long,

I'd have taken better care of myself.

—Sammy Davis, Jr.

When you rank exercise high, fitting it in gets easy. You do whatever it takes. You plan ahead, anticipate, rearrange your schedule, and postpone or cancel less important matters. When exercise is a priority in your life, time is no longer an issue.

However, you won't make physical activity a priority simply because I suggest it. You might begin to give it more importance if you do the following:

• **Schedule a physical exam.** If it has been awhile since you have exercised or had a check-up, call your doctor now and make an appointment. Your doctor will probably give you the green light to exercise.

On the other hand, if you receive a bit of bad news — you have high blood pressure or high cholesterol — your doctor will most likely prescribe exercise to help you improve your condition. Now you have added incentive to get fit.

If I spent as much time doing the things I worry
about as I do worrying about doing them,
I wouldn't have anything to worry about.

—Beryl Pfizer

• **Be moved by other people's misfortune.** If a friend or loved one is stricken with a life-threatening disease caused by poor health habits, picture yourself in that person's shoes. Visualize a typical day in your life if you had the same condition.

What would your next month be like? How about the rest of your life?

Appreciate the health you have and remind yourself how

you can strengthen your defense against numerous diseases and ailments by staying physically active.

• **Gain inspiration from elderly examples.** Are you looking for additional motivation to get you going? Take the time to admire people who lead active lives in their seventies, eighties and beyond, and you might decide to toss your excuses aside forever.

Aging athletes are all around us — in the gyms, on the hiking trails, in community-sponsored races and fun events. Look for them and draw strength from their accomplishments. Meanwhile, here are a few of my favorite examples. May their remarkable stories get you moving.

Hulda Crooks started hiking when she was in her sixties, shortly after her husband passed away. During the next twenty years, she hiked Mount Whitney, the highest peak in the contiguous United States, over twenty times.

At the age of eighty-nine, she hiked Mt. Fuji in Japan. The last I heard, Hulda was preparing to hike Mt. Kilimanjaro, the highest peak on the African continent.

Irene does aerobics three days a week, swims three times

a week, dances two nights a week, walks her dog every day and claims that she never gets tired. She stands under five feet, but appears tall because of her perfect posture.

At eighty-seven, Irene finds old people disgusting. In her words, "Their days are spent anticipating their next doctor's visit so they can get more prescription medication. That's all they do, and they're always miserable."

When Irene and I were trading goodbyes at the end of her two-week stay at the spa, she said, "If you're ever up my way, stop by for a visit. My name's in the phone book."

She turned to walk away, stopped abruptly, spun around and added, "Oh, but next June wouldn't be a good time. I'll be rafting the Colorado River through the Grand Canyon."

As long as you have a pulse, it is not too late to start moving your body.

—JS

At sixty-eight, Frank White was a smoker who suffered from heart disease, osteoarthritis, high blood pressure, high cholesterol and obesity. Finally, he took charge of his life, quit smoking, improved his diet and immersed himself in yoga. Over time, Frank's blood pressure returned to normal without medication, his cholesterol dropped from 400 to 150. He lost body fat, gained muscle and developed amazing flexibility for a man of any age. At seventy-five, Frank is leading students fifty years younger through rigorous Ashtanga yoga workouts.

At seventy-five, Herman Hoffer pedaled a bicycle over 3,000 miles across America. One year later, he did it again. At the age of eighty, accompanied by two "youngsters" in their sixties, Herman attempted his third cross-country bicycle journey. That year he made it 1,300 miles.

Several years after I first heard about Herman Hoffer, I saw him at a summer gathering of cross-country cyclists. I eagerly walked over and introduced myself to the bicycle legend who was now ninety-one years young and sporting a long white beard. Just to make conversation, I asked Herman if he still rides bicycles. I was not expecting an affirmative answer, but Herman proudly exclaimed, "I've ridden 1,800 miles so far this year."

• **Focus on what's important.** Examine what you really want to achieve with the rest of your life. Think about what you want to accomplish with your family, your business and your own being. How much more valuable will you be to others if you take care of yourself first?

• **Get started.** Your best chance of making exercise a priority occurs when you experience the benefits firsthand. Go ahead, get moving and see what the fuss is all about. You may have more questions today about fitness than you did yesterday, but you know enough to get started.

Apply the 24-10-30 Approach™

Motivation gets you going,
but habit gets you there.

—Zig Ziglar

24-10-30™ is not a locker combination. It's an effective strategy for forming a lifelong habit of fitness. Within the next **24** hours, devote **10** minutes to planning your exercise for the next **30** days. What exactly does this mean?

• **24** — Getting started within the next twenty-four hours is crucial. How many times have you failed to take action on a good idea because you didn't take action right away? If you don't start within twenty-four hours, you probably never will.

• **10** — Ten minutes is do-able. No matter how busy you are, you can find the time for a ten-minute effort. This concentrated ten minutes of planning will jump-start your fitness for the next thirty days — and hopefully for the rest of your life.

• **30** — Commit to thirty days of exercise. You need not work out every day, but consistency is the key. Thirty days is significant because it's enough time for you to form a habit.

Once, I broke my ankle and spent a

During your ten-minute commitment, permit no interruptions. If the phone rings, ignore it. Tell your spouse, children or cat that you will be busy for the next 600 seconds.

month on crutches. After my ankle healed and I was able to walk again, I instinctively reached for the crutches anyway whenever I intended to move. This lasted for several days. Walking with crutches had become a habit.

If, in thirty days, I can make walking with crutches feel natural, then in thirty days you can make physical activity feel natural.

No matter how sedentary you have been in the past, **24-10-30**™ is a powerful combination — but only if you use it. What are your plans for the next twenty-four hours?

You can't make footprints in the sands of time
if you're sitting on your butt.
And who wants to make buttprints
in the sands of time?

—Bob Moawad

Your Ten-Minute Solution™

Before you turn the page, complete the following:

✔ **Use the 24-10-30 Approach™ right now.**

- **Spend the next ten minutes deciding how you will be active during the next thirty days.**

- **Be realistic,** be specific, and put your plans on paper.

- **Vary your routine** to keep it fun and interesting.

Your Cool-Down

If we spent one-tenth the time doing health

that we spend talking about doing health,

we would all be reasonably fit individuals.

—JS

As you enter your cool-down phase, shift gears and reflect on how you have used this book so far. Have you read it in an active manner? Have you completed the assignments at the end of each step? Is your exercise program underway?

Your best chance for fitness success occurs when you incorporate all seven steps into your life. Think of them as the spokes on a bicycle wheel. If all seven spokes are in place, your wheel is strong. If even one spoke is missing, the other six are stressed and the integrity of your wheel is threatened. You might reach your destination on six or possibly five spokes, but why take the chance with something so essential to the quality of your life? Keep your wheel at maximum strength with every spoke firmly in place.

Your Final Assignment

Review each step and see if you are putting them in practice. Answer each question *yes* or *no*.

If you answer *yes* to all questions, congratulations! You are leading an active life.

If you answer *yes* to one question in each category, you are gaining some value from each step.

If you answer *no* to all questions within a category, you are avoiding that step.

Step 1. Make Exercise Fun

❑ Yes ❑ No   Are you doing physical activities you enjoy?

❑ Yes ❑ No   Do you vary your exercise often (duration, intensity or type of activity)?

❑ Yes ❑ No   Do you tune into how you feel during and right after a workout?

❏ Yes ❏ No   Have you removed the bathroom scale from your life?

❏ Yes ❏ No   Have you shifted your efforts from losing weight to gaining health?

Step 2. Give Pace A Chance

❏ Yes ❏ No   Are you patient with your fitness progress?

❏ Yes ❏ No   Do you see value in a ten-minute walk?

❏ Yes ❏ No   If you are a beginner, are you using the **10-15-20**™ approach?

Step 3. Plan To Move

❏ Yes ❏ No   Do you write down your exercise plans in red ink?

❏ Yes ❏ No   Are you aiming to achieve a long-range exercise goal within three or six months?

❏ Yes ❏ No   Did you work out consistently during your last business or pleasure trip?

❏ Yes ❏ No   Are you planning a way to keep physically active during November and December?

Step 4. Gather Support

❏ Yes ❏ No   Do you have one or two regular workout partners?

❏ Yes ❏ No   Do you pay ahead for a block of exercise classes?

❏ Yes ❏ No   Do you propose active gatherings with friends and business colleagues? Have you organized a hike-a-month club?

❏ Yes ❏ No   Have you been **Netwalking**™ lately?

Step 5. Balance Your Workouts

❏ Yes ❏ No   Do you elevate your heartrate for at least fifteen to twenty minutes, three days a week?

❏ Yes ❏ No   Do you do at least ten minutes of strength training on two to three non-consecutive days a week?

❏ Yes ❏ No   Do all your workouts include a warm-up and a cool-down?

❏ Yes ❏ No   Do you end every workout with five to ten minutes of stretching?

❑ Yes ❑ No   Do you always exercise in your comfort zone and stop if you feel pain?

❑ Yes ❑ No   Have you identified the weak link(s) in your exercise program?

❑ Yes ❑ No   Are you regularly working your weaknesses?

Step 6. Take Active Vacations

❑ Yes ❑ No   In the past six months, have you experienced, or at least scheduled, an active vacation?

❑ Yes ❑ No   Have you requested catalogs from at least three active outfits listed in the appendix?

❑ Yes ❑ No   Have you called your active-minded friends to hear details of their most recent adventures?

Step 7. Make Exercise A Priority

❑ Yes ❑ No   Do you constantly look ahead for ways to fit in a little exercise here and there?

❑ Yes ❑ No   Do you have an exercise gear bag packed and stored at work or in your car?

❏ Yes ❏ No   When a friend suggests lunch, do you recommend a walk, followed by lunch?

❏ Yes ❏ No   Do you remind yourself often that if you don't take care of yourself, you can't take care of your family or your career?

If you have taken little or no action so far, don't beat yourself up over it. Just get on track by flipping through the book again. Find a simple idea for each step that will work for you. Plenty of easy-to-implement ideas are waiting for you. Get started now and you will get moving for life.

It's amazing how often people put things off when the solution to their predicament is at their fingertips.

One day while showering, I noticed the flow of water was less than normal. I thought "Hmm, I'd better get that fixed," but I took no action—for two weeks. Finally, I altered my usual routine when I stepped into the tub. Before turning on the water, I unscrewed the showerhead fixture, removed a small disc from inside, tapped the disc against the shower wall and watched a few grains of sand fall out of the tiny holes in the disc. I reinserted the disc, reattached the showerhead, turned on the water and felt a strong spray of water on my body.

For two weeks, I did nothing to correct my situation. When I finally took action, I fixed the problem in less than one minute.

In only one minute, you can take a giant step to moving again. You can't get fit in a minute, but in 60 seconds you can call a potential workout partner or request information on an active vacation or complete the first minute of a ten-minute walk.

Have you been feeling stressed or sluggish lately? Are your clothes fitting tighter? Exercise can cure many of your ills. Are you ready to get moving?

Have you got a minute?

Just Start.

—JS

Afterword

I welcome your comments. Let me know what ideas from this book have worked best for you, what hasn't worked and how this book can be improved.

Describe how your life, exercise-wise, is different now and how you feel as a result of it.

Finally, when you take an active vacation, send me a postcard!

Enjoy your journey in health,

Joe Sweeney

P.O. Box 927915

San Diego, CA 92192-7915

APPENDIX

Recommended Resources For Active Vacations

Backroads
1-800-462-2848
Bicycling, walking
& hiking trips

Bicycling Magazine
Rodale Press, Inc.
33 E. Minor Street
Emmaus, PA 18098
1-800-848-4735

Canoe & Kayaking Magazine
PO Box 7011
Red Oak, IA 51591
1-800-678-5432

Earthwatch
PO Box 403
Watertown, MA 02272
1-800-776-0188
Environmental expeditions;
non-profit; connects
volunteers with ongoing
research projects

EcoTraveler
PO Box 469003
Escondido, CA 92046
1-800-334-8152

Escape Magazine
PO Box 5159
Santa Monica, CA 90409
310-392-5235
Adventure travel

Natural History Magazine
American Museum
of Natural History
Central Park West
at 79th Street
New York, NY 10024
1-800-234-5252

Rivers & Oceans
PO Box 40321
Flagstaff, AZ 86004
1-800-473-4576
A travel company
and source for river trips
in the Grand Canyon

Outdoor Photographer
Magazine
Box 57213
Boulder, CO 80322
1-800-283-4410
Photographic travel
and workshops

Sierra Magazine
Sierra Club
85 Second Street
San Francisco, CA 94105-3441
415-977-5653
Adventures by foot, bicycle,
sea kayak, raft, skis & more

Smithsonian Magazine
Smithsonian Associates
900 Jefferson Drive
Washington, DC 20560
1-800-766-2149

The Spa Finder
91 Fifth Avenue, Suite #301
New York, NY 10003-3039
1-800-255-7727
Catalog of spas,
fitness resorts & retreats

TravelFit
Prestige Publications, Inc.
4151 Knob Drive
Eagan, MN 55122

University Research
Expeditions Program
University of California
Berkeley, CA 94720-7050
510-642-6586
Environmental expeditions;
connects volunteers with
ongoing research projects

The Walking Magazine
PO Box 56561
Boulder, CO 80322
1-800-678-0881

Books

Growing Old
Is Not For Sissies
Pomegranate Calendars
& Books
1-800-227-1428
Inspiring stories & photos
of aging athletes

Walden
A classic
by Henry David Thoreau

Newsletter

University of California at
Berkeley Wellness Letter
904-445-6414
Newsletter on wellness

If you're interested in having Joe Sweeney speak

or conduct a workshop

for your company or organization,

call (619) 452-3059

or toll-free in the USA

1-800-700-5088.

Give yourself, your friends and your loved ones the best gift of all — the gift of health! Order Joe Sweeney's book and audio cassette tapes.

Stretch, Tone & Relax with Joe Sweeney

Side 1: Total Body Stretches .... 34 minutes

Progressive Relaxation .... 11 minutes

Side 2: Toning Exercises for Abdominals & Backs .... 20 minutes

Standing Stretches (a post-exercise stretch routine) .... 13 minutes

How to Fit a Healthy Life Into a Busy Life

Side 1: Live Presentation .... 30 minutes

Side 2: Fitness Tips for the Road .... 25 minutes

Mail this order form with check payable to:

Pacific Valley Press
PO Box 927915
San Diego, CA 92192-7915

Quantity	Title	Unit Price	Total
	Stretch, Tone & Relax with Joe Sweeney (tape)	$10.00	
	How to Fit a Healthy Life Into a Busy Life (tape)	$10.00	
	I Know I Should Exercise, But… (book)	$14.95	
	Subtotal		
	CA residents, please add 7.75% sales tax		
	Shipping/Handling: $1.00 per tape		
	Shipping/Handling: $3.00 for first book and $2.00 per additional book		
	TOTAL		

Please ship my order to:

Name _____

Address _____

City _____ State _____Zip _____

Phone (_____) _____ ❑ Home ❑ Work

Give yourself, your friends and your loved ones the best gift of all — the gift of health! Order Joe Sweeney's book and audio cassette tapes.

Stretch, Tone & Relax with Joe Sweeney

Side 1:	Total Body Stretches	34 minutes
	Progressive Relaxation	11 minutes
Side 2:	Toning Exercises for Abdominals & Backs	20 minutes
	Standing Stretches (a post-exercise stretch routine)	13 minutes

How to Fit a Healthy Life Into a Busy Life

Side 1:	Live Presentation	30 minutes
Side 2:	Fitness Tips for the Road	25 minutes

Mail this order form with check payable to:

Pacific Valley Press
PO Box 927915
San Diego, CA 92192-7915

Quantity	Title	Unit Price	Total
	Stretch, Tone & Relax with Joe Sweeney (tape)	$10.00	
	How to Fit a Healthy Life Into a Busy Life (tape)	$10.00	
	I Know I Should Exercise, But... (book)	$14.95	
	Subtotal		
	CA residents, please add 7.75% sales tax		
	Shipping/Handling: $1.00 per tape		
	Shipping/Handling: $3.00 for first book and $2.00 per additional book		
	TOTAL		

Please ship my order to:

Name _____

Address _____

City _____ State _____ Zip _____

Phone (_____) _____ ❑ Home ❑ Work